Substance and Non Substance Related Addiction Disorders: Diagnosis and Treatment

Edited by:

Subhash C. Bhatia

Department of Psychiatry, Mental Health and Behavioral Sciences, Creighton University; Department VA Nebraska- Western Iowa Health Care System, Omaha, NE, USA

Co-Editors:

Frederick Petty

Department of Psychiatry, Creighton University; VA Nebraska Western Iowa Health Care System Orlando VA Medical Center, Orlando, Florida, USA

&

Teri Gabel

VA Nebraska Western Iowa Health Care System, Clinical Pharmacy Specialist - Mental Health; Department of Psychiatry, University of Nebraska College of Medicine Omaha NE 68198; Drug Therapy Consultants, Omaha NE, USA

Bentham Science Publishers Ltd.
Executive Suite Y - 2
PO Box 7917, Saif Zone
Sharjah, U.A.E.
Email: subscriptions@benthamscience.org

CONTENTS

FOREWORD

About one person in three has a problem with potentially hazardous drug or alcohol use which often goes unrecognized. Excessive or hazardous use of drugs, including tobacco, and of alcohol, can have very negative biological, psychological and socio-economic consequences from the direct effect of the substances. In social realm addictive behaviors take a toll on relationships with friends and family. Also often harm can occur to the patient by failure to comply with medical or psychosocial treatment for abstinence or unsupervised withdrawal or through drug interactions. Thus, every practitioner should have knowledge regarding diagnosis and treatment of common substance use disorders.

The authors share with the readers wealth of information based on their experience about diagnosis and management of common substances of abuse as well as neurobiological underpinning of these disorders. Each chapter in section II features discussion of diagnosis, and approaches to treatment and highlights cases with approaches to the patient delineated.

The practitioners should find this volume useful, helpful, and interesting in helping to provide optimal health care to his or her patients.

Frederick Petty
Department of Psychiatry
Creighton University
VA Nebraska Western Iowa Health Care System
Orlando VA Medical Center
Orlando, Florida
USA

PREFACE

Substance use disorders are amongst the major causes of disease burden around the globe. In a World Drug Report by the United Nations Office on Drug and Crime it is estimated that 210 million individuals have used illicit drugs at least once and that these drugs are related to about 200,000 deaths. The economic burden of substance use disorders in the USA alone from health care costs, lost productivity, crime, incarceration and drug enforcement is estimated to be $524 billion.

Addiction is a brain disease where a person uses a drug compulsively despite negative consequences and drug use in turn causes persistent changes in the brain circuits which perpetuates its use. In predisposed individual's addiction starts during adolescent years. Fortunately addictions are preventable through public awareness and education and are treatable through contemporary medications, individual, group or family therapy as a well as self-help groups. Biopsychosocial intervention can mitigate life time suffering of the patient, family, and friends. Treatment also improves the quality of their lives. Moreover it can prevent tragic loss of life as well . Extended abstinence predicts long-term recovery. Drug addiction is a chronic disease and its relapse rate is comparable to hypertension, diabetes or asthma.

Recently one notable development has been publication of DSM-5 . Our publication provides information on the diagnosis of the additive disorders consistent with this new version of DSM.

The book is titled *Substance and Non Substance Related Addiction Disorders: Diagnosis and Treatment* and is divided in to three sections.

Section I addresses basic general topics related to scientific underpinnings of addictive disorders including the neurobiology and addiction neural reward pathways, genetics and psychosocial basis of addictions; urine drug screens in diagnosis and management of substance use disorders, co-occurring psychiatric and substance use disorders and pharmacological treatment of comorbid psychiatric disorders and motivational interviewing. Each chapter has key learning points, references, a patient education hand out .

Section II provides updated information about individual drug related addictive disorder. Each chapter in addition to key learning points and a patient education handout, describes a case vignette and its discussion related to specific drug, its diagnosis, medical and biopsychosocial interventions. In addition these chapters include neurobiology, epidemiology summary and updated references with resources for more information.

Section III presents information about non-substance related addiction disorders, a vignette and its discussion, diagnosis and interdisciplinary treatment strategies. The chapter in this section is primarily devoted to gambling addiction; other non-substance related addictions are also mentioned.

This book is by multiple authors with experience in addictions and is designed to meet the clinical practice needs of internists, family physicians, nurse practitioners, physician assistants, addiction therapists, psychiatry and primary care residents, graduate students and other health care professionals interested in the care of patients with substance use and addiction disorders. A concise format for each chapter is used to maintain its user friendliness for quick review.

Subhash C. Bhatia
Department of Psychiatry
Mental Health and Behavioral Sciences
Creighton University; Department VA Nebraska- Western
Iowa Health Care System , Omaha, NE, USA
&
Frederick Petty
Department of Psychiatry
Creighton University
VA Nebraska Western Iowa Health Care System
Orlando VA Medical Center
Orlando, Florida
USA
&
Teri Gabel
VA Nebraska Western Iowa Health Care System
Clinical Pharmacy Specialist - Mental Health
Department of Psychiatry
University of Nebraska College of Medicine, Omaha NE 68198
Drug Therapy Consultants
Omaha NE USA

List of Contributors

Aly Hassan	Phoenix VA Health Care System, Department of Psychiatry, University of Arizona, Phoenix College of Medicine, Gilbert VA Clinic, 3285 S Val Vista Drive, Gilbert, AZ 85925, USA
Frederick Petty	Orlando VA Medical Center, Orlando, Florida, USA Orange City Community Based Outpatient Clinic, 2583 South Volusia Ave #300, Orange City, Florida 32763, USA
Imad Alsakaf	Creighton University School of Medicine, 3528 Dodge Street, Omaha, USA
James Meyer	Inroads to Recovery, 2808 N 75th ST, Omaha, NE 68134, USA
Jayakrishna S. Madabushi	Baptist Health System, 517, Crowne Woods Drive, Birmingham, AL 35244, USA
Prasad R. Padala	Clinical, VISN 16 Geriatric Research Education and Clinical Center (GRECC), Deaprtment of Psychiatry and Geriatrics, UAMS, 2200 Fort Roots Drive, North Little Rock, AR 72114, USA
R. Dario Pulido	Mental Health and Behavioral Sciences, Department VA Nebraska-Western Iowa Health Care System, 4101 Woolworth Ave., Omaha, NE 68105, USA
Shashi K. Bhatia	Departments of Psychiatry and Pediatrics, Division of Child and Adolescent Psychiatry, Creighton University, 3528 Dodge, Omaha NE 68131, USA
Sidney Kauzlarich	Douglas County Community Mental Health Center, 4102 Woolworth Ave, Omaha, NE 68105, USA
Subhash C. Bhatia	Department of Psychiatry, Mental Health and Behavioral Sciences, Creighton University; Department VA Nebraska- Western Iowa Health Care System 4101 Woolworth Ave, Omaha, NE 68105, USA
Teri Gabel	VA Nebraska Western Iowa Health Care System, Clinical Pharmacy Specialist - Mental Health, Omaha, NE 68105; Department of Psychiatry, University Of Nebraska College of Medicine, Omaha, NE 68198, USA Drug Therapy Consultants, PC 5116 N 116 St, Omaha, NE 68164, USA
Usha Kanthety	Staff Physician, CHI, 1721, Colfax St, Schuyler, NE 68661, USA
Venkata Kolli	Child and Adolescent Fellowship Training Program, Department of Psychiatry, Creighton University School of Medicine, 3528 Dodge Street Omaha, NE 68131, USA
Vidhyalakshmi Selvaraj	Department of Psychiatry, Creighton University, 3528 Dodge, Omaha, NE 68131, USA

This book is dedicated to our Teachers, Parents and Persons with Substance use Disorders.

CHAPTER 1

Neurobiology and Psycho-Social Basis for Addiction and Related Disorders

Subhash C. Bhatia*

Department of Psychiatry, Mental Health and Behavioral Sciences, Creighton University; Department VA Nebraska- Western Iowa Health Care System 4101 Woolworth Ave Omaha, NE 68105, USA

Abstract: Addictive disorders are diseases of the brain. Addictions like chronic illness may have remissions and relapses. These are caused by genetic, biological, psychological, social and economic factors. Reward pathways for all substance and non-substance related addictive behavior (gambling, sex and food addiction *etc.*) are similar and are mediated through nucleus accumbens and associated circuits. Negative preexisting emotional state or due to withdrawal from substance and self-medication to seek relief may perpetuate addictive behavior. Substance or non-substance related addictive behavior-pleasure-reinforcement-reuse paradigm perpetuates addictive behavior. Environmental cues and memories associated with addiction related activities contribute to craving and relapse. Dopamine neurotransmitter plays major role in addictive behaviors. Treatment consideration should factor in all of these biopsychosocial factors.

Keywords: Addiction reward pathways, Cues and craving, Dopamine, Nucleus accumbens, Operant conditioning, Self-medication theory.

KEY LEARNING POINTS

1. Addictive disorders have complex biopsychosocial underpinnings for both causation and treatment.

* **Corresponding author Subhash C. Bhatia:** Department of Psychiatry, Mental Health and Behavioral Sciences, Creighton University; Department VA Nebraska- Western Iowa Health Care System 4101 Woolworth Ave Omaha, NE 68105, USA; Tel/Fax: (402)-995-4315/(402)-995-4240; Email: sub55@cox.net

2. Dopamine is the crucial neurotransmitter in reward circuits for all substance and non-substance related addictive disorders. Chronic use causes down regulation of dopamine receptors which accounts for tolerance.
3. Ventral tegmental area, nucleus accumbens, prefrontal cortex, hippocampus, amygdala and basal ganglia all contribute to impulsive and compulsive drug use as well as reward and cue driven craving.
4. Psychosocial stressors as epigenetic factor may change the genotype and may increase propensity to addiction.
5. Association of behaviors leading to reward is part of the operant conditioning paradigm and perpetuates drug use.
6. The self-medication hypothesis to treat negative emotional states is reported to be involved with addiction.
7. Adverse childhood experiences such as physical, sexual, emotional abuse, physical or emotional neglect, domestic violence and drug misuse or mental illness in the family, incarceration of a family member and parental separation and divorce may increase the risk of illicit drug use 2 to 4 times. This drug use may be viewed as self-soothing behavior and may persist through life.

NEUROBIOLOGY OF ADDICTION AND REWARD PATHWAYS

The neurobiology of substance and non-substance addiction and related disorders is complex but follows a common reward pathway. These disorders are chronic relapsing illnesses, a brain disease, characterized by engaging in the compulsive use of substances despite negative consequences. The drug use starts out with liking, which is a non-problematic use, followed by wanting and craving respectively leading to abuse and dependence. The intense craving is mediated by withdrawal effects, or after due to pleasurable effects of drug and/or environmental cues. The motivation to repeatedly re-experiencing pleasurable effects or to avoid aversive effects of drug withdrawal [1, 2]. This compels the individual to seek the drug. The following information provides a simplified summary version using an example of narcotic addiction.

For addictions, self-administration mimics binding of a substance directly to specific endogenous receptors resulting in reinforcing effects. For example in opiate addiction mu receptor activation in addition to causing analgesia, nausea, reduced bowel motility, miosis (constricted pupils), sedation, reduced blood pressure and decreased respiration is also associated with euphoria [3]. Both substance and behavioral addictions are mediated through dopamine (DA) neurotransmission. DA is a primary neurotransmitter in reward pathways. DA is also responsible for emotion, cognition, motivation and euphoria and dysregulation of reward pathways and is considered the cause for addiction [4]. The dopamine neurotransmission is basis for addiction and related disorders through mesocortocolimbic dopamine projections from the ventral tegmental area (VTA) to the nucleus accumbens (NAc) [5].

Acute positive reinforcement, euphoria or the "high" is through the effect of DA and local opioid peptides through the common reward pathways *i.e.* VTA to nucleus accumbens (NAc) - amygdala reward system (5). Repeated replication of this positive reinforcement forms the basis of addiction.

Chronic substance use leads to neuroadaptation through decreased VTA mesolimbic and NAc DA neurotransmission [6]. Repeated use and excessive production of dopamine leads to down regulation of dopamine receptor sites. To experience the same level of euphoria again, an individual needs higher amounts. This forms the basis for tolerance. Also, stress results in increased production of corticotrophin releasing factor (CRF). This activates the hypothalamic-pituitar--adrenal axis (HPA) and other stress system like the amygdala [7]. This forms the basis for negative emotional states like dysphoria and anxiety. Individuals use substances to deal with these negative emotional states which promote addictive process. CRF adaptation may also explain role of stress and emotional states in craving for drug use (6).

Dysfunction of ventro-medial prefrontal cortex circuitry is the cause for impulsivity expressed as a sense of urgency, lack of evaluative and rational decision making processes [8]. This contributes to impulsive drug use.

Environmental cue-induced craving is mediated through hippocampus and basolateral amygdala [6].

The compulsive drug-seeking behavior is hypothesized to be driven by ventral striatal-ventral pallidum-thalamic-cortical loops [7]. Drug seeking behavior despite harmful consequences may point towards impairment of executive functions.

Treatment directed at craving, stress modulation, promotion of resilience in dealing with stress and impulse control through cognitive behavior therapy is a valuable intervention for all substance and non-substance related addictive behaviors.

PSYCHOSOCIAL FACTORS

Genetic factors and heritability account for 40-60% of the risk for addictive disorders. Environmental factors may contribute to the change in brain circuits during development which may further contribute to susceptibility of individuals to drug use. Animal studies have shown that stress can contribute to changes in genotype [9].

The self- medication hypothesis postulates that some individuals abuse substances to deal with intolerable emotional states of mind [10]. For example patients with depression may prefer stimulants to relieve symptoms or patients with anxiety may prefer alcohol, a self-directed therapy for anxiety. Patients crave to reuse a drug to seek relief from these dysphoric emotional states.

Drug seeking and drug intake behavior and its association with euphoria, reinforcement and reward are components of operant conditioning which plays a part in addiction

Socio-economic factors like poverty and their impact on social development have a strong association with addiction [11]. These factors also contribute to stress and self-medication is probably one way to seek relief from it. It is also postulated that “drugs are more likely to be a consequence of poverty and crime” [12].

Lastly, social factors such as peer pressure and the easy availability of a drug in a community play a role in addiction and related disorders.

ADVERSE CHILDHOOD EXPERIENCES (ACE)

Children who experience physical, sexual, emotional abuse, physical or emotional neglect, domestic violence and drug misuse or mental illness in the family, incarceration of a family member and parental separation and divorce experience chronic stressful events which has negative impact on multiple biopsychosocial functional domains. These childhood disruptions cause neurodevelopment disruptions, depression, interpersonal and family dysfunction, cognitive impairment, early engagement in high risk behaviors, smoking, consuming alcohol, abusing prescription and illicit drugs, engaging in risky sexual behaviors during teen age years as well as afflicted with disease disability and premature mortality [13]. Substance use is often a coping mechanism to deal with emotional pain. Substance use related effects are dose-response *i.e.* proportionate to degree and severity of adversity. Each adverse experiences increases the risk of early initiation of illicit drug use. There is 2-4 times risk of initiation in to early illicit drug use. Addictive behaviors often start with early initiation of alcohol [14], early smoking initiation [15] and prescription drug use [16]. These addictive behaviors may continue in to adulthood and even may persist through lifetime [17, 18]. Dose related effects of adverse childhood events may also include lifetime depressive episodes [19] and risk of suicide attempts, sleep disturbances [20], high risk sexual behaviors and teen pregnancy [21]. Depression and sleep disturbances may further compound substance use. Surveillance and data acquisition about ACE, increasing awareness with state and county, developing programs, policies and processes for early intervention and prevention planning are valuable.

CONFLICT OF INTEREST

The author confirms that he has no conflict of interest to declare for this publication.

ACKNOWLEDGEMENTS

Declared none.

REFERENCES

[1] Wikler A. Recent progress in research on the neurophysiologic basis of morphine addiction. Am J Psychiatry 1948; 105(5): 329-38.
[http://dx.doi.org/10.1176/ajp.105.5.329] [PMID: 18890902]

[2] Koob GF, Stinus L, Le Moal M, Bloom FE. Opponent process theory of motivation: neurobiological evidence from studies of opiate dependence. Neurosci Biobehav Rev 1989; 13(2-3): 135-40. [http://dx.doi.org/10.1016/S0149-7634(89)80022-3] [PMID: 2682399]

[3] http://en.wikipedia.org/wiki/Mu_Opiod_receptor 2010.

[4] Koob G, Kreek MJ. Stress, dysregulation of drug reward pathways, and the transition to drug dependence. Am J Psychiatry 2007; 164(8): 1149-59. [http://dx.doi.org/10.1176/appi.ajp.2007.05030503] [PMID: 17671276]

[5] Koob GF, Sanna PP, Bloom FE. Neuroscience of addiction. Neuron 1998; 21(3): 467-76. [http://dx.doi.org/10.1016/S0896-6273(00)80557-7] [PMID: 9768834]

[6] Koob GF, Simon EJ. The Neurobiology of addiction: where we have been and where we are going. J Drug Issues 2009; 39(1): 115-32. [http://dx.doi.org/10.1177/002204260903900110] [PMID: 20622969]

[7] Sarnyai Z, Shaham Y, Heinrichs SC. The role of corticotropin-releasing factor in drug addiction. Pharmacol Rev 2001; 53(2): 209-43. [PMID: 11356984]

[8] Brewer JA, Potenza MN. The neurobiology and genetics of impulse control disorders: relationships to drug addictions. Biochem Pharmacol 2008; 75(1): 63-75. [http://dx.doi.org/10.1016/j.bcp.2007.06.043] [PMID: 17719013]

[9] Kendler KS, Neale MC, Heath AC, Kessler RC, Eaves LJ. A twin-family study of alcoholism in women. Am J Psychiatry 1994; 151(5): 707-15. [http://dx.doi.org/10.1176/ajp.151.5.707] [PMID: 8166312]

[10] Khantzian EJ. The self-medication hypothesis of addictive disorders: focus on heroin and cocaine dependence. Am J Psychiatry 1985; 142(11): 1259-64. [http://dx.doi.org/10.1176/ajp.142.11.1259] [PMID: 3904487]

[11] Galea S, Nandi A, Vlahov D. The social epidemiology of substance use. Epidemiol Rev 2004; 26: 36-52. [http://dx.doi.org/10.1093/epirev/mxh007] [PMID: 15234946]

[12] Hart C. High Price: A neuroscientist's journey of self-discovery that challenges everything you know about drugs and society. HarperCollins 2013.

[13] http://en.wikipedia.org/wiki/Mu_Opiod_receptor

[14] Dube SR, Miller JW, Brown DN. Adverse childhood experiences and association with ever using alcohol and early initiating alcohol use during adolescents. J Adolesc Health 2006; 38(444): 1-10. [PMID: 16387241]

[15] Anda RF, Croft JB, Felitti VJ, *et al.* Adverse childhood experiences and smoking during adolescence and adulthood. JAMA 1999; 282(17): 1652-8. [http://dx.doi.org/10.1001/jama.282.17.1652] [PMID: 10553792]

[16] Anda RF, Brown DW, Felitti VJ, Dube SR, Giles WH. Adverse childhood experiences and prescription drug use in a cohort study of adult HMO patients. BMC Public Health 2008; 8: 198. [http://dx.doi.org/10.1186/1471-2458-8-198] [PMID: 18533034]

[17] Dube SR, Anda RF, Felitti VJ, Edwards VJ, Croft JB. Adverse childhood experiences and personal alcohol abuse as an adult. Addict Behav 2002; 27(5): 713-25. [http://dx.doi.org/10.1016/S0306-4603(01)00204-0] [PMID: 12201379]

[18] Ford ES, Anda RF, Edwards VJ, *et al.* Adverse childhood experiences and smoking status in five states. Prev Med 2011; 53(3): 188-93. [http://dx.doi.org/10.1016/j.ypmed.2011.06.015] [PMID: 21726575]

[19] Chapman DP, Whitfield CL, Felitti VJ, Dube SR, Edwards VJ, Anda RF, *et al.* Adverse childhood experiences and the risk of depressive disorder in adulthood. J Affect Disord 2008; 84: 217-25.

[20] Chapman DP, Wheaton AG, Anda RF, *et al.* Adverse childhood experiences and sleep disturbances in adults. Sleep Med 2011; 12(8): 773-9. [http://dx.doi.org/10.1016/j.sleep.2011.03.013] [PMID: 21704556]

[21] Hillis SD, Anda RF, Dube SR, Felitti VJ, Marchbanks PA, Marks JS. The association between adverse childhood experiences and adolescent pregnancy, long-term psychosocial consequences, and fetal death. Pediatrics 2004; 113(2): 320-7. [http://dx.doi.org/10.1542/peds.113.2.320] [PMID: 14754944]

CHAPTER 2

Urine Drug Screening (UDS) in the Management of Substance Use Disorders

Teri Gabel*

VA Nebraska Western Iowa Health Care System, Clinical Pharmacy Specialist - Mental Health, Omaha, NE 68105; Department of Psychiatry, University Of Nebraska College of Medicine Omaha NE 68198; Drug Therapy Consultants, PC 5116 N 116 St, Omaha NE 68164 USA

Abstract: Urine drug screens can add accountability to a patient's recovery plan. An upfront discussion of the role of the urine drug screen in treatment is important for a solid provider client therapeutic relationship. Substance use disorders are relapsing and remitting disorders. The goal of treatment is to extend the duration of sobriety until it is life-long, a lifestyle. The role of the urine drug screen in a treatment program should be therapeutic not penalizing. Understanding what a drug screen can and can not do in providing information is important. Using a consistent screen and appropriately certified laboratory is a must. This chapter covers the types of drug screens, the substances identified in a standard urine dug screen and provides guidance on when other substances may need to be requested during screening. Some substances such as "bath salts" are not identified in current urine drug screens. In clinical situations it will be important to confirm any positive results found on a urine drug screen. Common agents and medications that cause false positive or negative results are identified in the chapter. Proper process for obtaining and handling the urine sample including proper chain of custody are presented.

Keywords: Adulteration, Bath salts, Chain of custody, False negative, False positive.

* **Corresponding author Teri Gabel:** VA Nebraska Western Iowa Health Care System, Clinical Pharmacy Specialist - Mental Health, Omaha, NE 68105; Department of Psychiatry, University Of Nebraska College of Medicine Omaha NE 68198; Drug Therapy Consultants, PC 5116 N 116 St, Omaha NE 68164 USA; Tel: 402 (493-5222); Email: pharmdherb@gmail.com

Subhash C. Bhatia (Ed.)

KEY LEARNING POINTS

1. Most urine drug screens test for 5 common agents *i.e.* amphetamines, cocaine, PCP, Opiates (codeine and morphine), marijuana. Other substances to be tested must be added to the test request.
2. Urine drug screens do not identify certain substances like "Bath Salts".
3. Urine drug screen positive results must be confirmed before their use in any clinical decision making.
4. Certain medications can interfere with the results of a urine drug screen.
5. For legal reasons chain of custody of obtained samples must be maintained.
6. Urine samples must be evaluated for pH, temperature, specific gravity and adulteration.
7. Know the issues regarding the urine drug screen performed at your facility – what is tested for routinely, what false positives may occur with the process utilized.

CLINICAL VIGNETTE

Charles works in a high stress job with a large company that has a random drug screening program. His most recent urine drug screen was positive for phencyclidine (PCP). Charles is in danger of being fired from his job. Looking at his medical record, Charles is being treated for high blood pressure, high cholesterol and anxiety. His medications are simvastatin, venlafaxine, propranolol and a multiple vitamin.

DIAGNOSTIC CONSIDERATION

In this patient a drug screen may have value for clinical management acutely and for follow up. A legal issue may also surface if this patient is actually fired. Charles is being treated with venlafaxine which can yield a false positive for PCP with some immunoassay urine screens. The confirmation test should verify the false positive. Based on that Charles would be in no danger of losing his job.

REASONS FOR OBTAINING AN UDS

1. Medical: UDS may be beneficial when the patient is presenting with unusual symptoms or acting in a strange fashion. In instances of emergency

presentation for overdose, seizure, or other situations a UDS can be of immense importance.

2. Legal: UDS may be required for employment, probation or other legal issues.
3. Therapeutic: UDS can assist in the clarification of a diagnosis as part of the work up of a differential diagnosis. Once diagnosed with a substance use disorder the use of urine drug screens can be useful in monitoring compliance with treatment and sobriety.

It is important to consider the reason for UDS and its usefulness as in the vignette above. It is interesting to note at times UDS adds a piece of the puzzle not a diagnostic conclusion [1].

Depending on the substance involved, the results of the UDS may impact treatment both in the acute and follow up phase. This may also provide a tool to help identify reasons for relapse from psychiatric illness or help correlate with triggers for reuse of illicit drugs.

With alcohol use disorders medications such as naltrexone and acamprosate may be continued in light of a confirmed positive urine drug screen for ethanol. Alcohol is not included in a routine UDS and must be requested in addition to the baseline urine drug screen. Should the UDS show positive for other substances, treatment may need to be adjusted to address the clinical needs of the patient.

When used with a narcotic treatment contract and contingency management the results of a confirmed positive or negative result for the opioid/opiate adds value to assist with sobriety from drugs. A positive UDS for another substance of abuse may result in termination of the narcotic agent depending on the contract. UDS for opioids are relatively unreliable, many do not test for the desired agent and like alcohol it is important to request they test for the specific agent being prescribed [4 - 6].

URINE DRUG SCREENS

It is recommended that urine drug screens be performed by a laboratory that is certified by the Department of Health and Human Services (DHHS). This guarantees the use of standardized testing processes and procedures to provide

consistent reliable and valid results.
(http://workplace.samhsa.gov/ResourceCenter/lablist.htm)

Urine assay allows for the presence or absence of certain drugs to be evaluated with (relatively) good specificity, sensitivity, ease of administration, and reasonable cost.

Types of Urine Drug Tests

Screens: Urine Drug Screens determine the presence or absence of particular substances according to predetermined threshold levels. Screens can be performed in either the office or at a laboratory. Urine drug screens are immunoassays. Immunoassays use antibodies to the substrate that combine with the substance of abuse causing a change (form a line or change color) in the test medium.

The two most common types of immunoassay screens are the Enzyme Multiplied Immunoassay (EMIT) and the Fluorescence Polarized Immunoassay (FPIA).

Office-based drug screens can be performed using one of the in office screening tests on the market. These screens use a urine "dip stick" to identify the presence of classes of substances in the urine. They have a different level of sensitivity compared to laboratory-based screening tests.

Screening tests generally have a higher cutoff and as a result it may be possible for a patient to have used a substance but the level in their urine is under that cut off number leading to a false negative report (Table **1**).

Confirmation Screens: A positive urine drug screen requires a confirmation screen. These identify the specific drug present *via* Gas Chromatography/Mass Spectroscopy (GC/MS) Thin Layer Chromatography (TLC), or High Performance Liquid Chromatography (HPLC). Confirmatory tests are done by an outside laboratory. Positive and negative tests are determined by established cut off levels for substances.

The cutoff amounts in confirmatory tests are much lower and would be able to detect this use if there were doubts about its being positive during the screen [1] (Table **1**).

Urine Drug Test as a Follow-up Tool

The timing of UDS should be random and irregular intervals for optimal usefulness. For substance use disorders testing is recommended randomly during the first 1-2 years of sobriety then annually or as clinically indicated.

Table 1. Time found in the urine and urinary cut off amounts.

Agent	Duration when UDS can be positive	Product tested for	Cut off UDS screen (ng/ml)	Cut off UDS confirmation (ng/ml)
Amphetamine	2-5 days	amphetamine	1,000	500
Barbiturates	short acting: 4 days long acting: up to 30 days	amobarbital secobarbital others	200	200
Benzodiazepines	up to 30 days depending on the half-life of the agent	oxazepam diazepam nordiazepam others	200	200
Cocaine	1-3 days heavy use up to 8 days	benzoylecgonine	300	150
Codeine	1-3 days	codeine morphine	300 300	300
Heroin	1-3 days	morphine 6 – acetylmorphine	300 10	300 10
Marijuana	periodic use: 1-5 days chronic use: up to 30 days	tetrahydrocannabinol	100 50 10	15
Methadone	2-4 days	methadone	300	300
Methamphetamine	2-4 days	methamphetamine amphetamine	1,000	500 200
Phencyclidine	periodic use: 2-7 days chronic use: up to 30 days	phencyclidine	25	25

Adapted from references [1, 5, 6]

Urine Sample Collection

Depending on the reason for the type of UDS, collection of the urine sample may be witnessed or un-witnessed. Any suspicious unobserved urine would necessitate the immediate recollection of a witnessed sample. The sample should be obtained in a special urine sample container which has indicators for pH and temperature at a minimum.

Chain of Custody

Securing the sample maintains credibility of the test result. This process is more important when testing is done for reasons of employment or legal issues.

Specific Criteria About Urine Samples: A urine specimen must meet certain criteria to provide a valid result.

1. Temperature: if collected within 4 minutes, the temperature range of urine should be between 90° and 100° F.
2. Urine pH should be between 4.5 and 8.
3. Creatinine norm is 20 mg/dl or greater. Diluted urine has <20 mg/dl creatinine, while urine with <5 mg/dl of creatinine is extremely dilute and may not be human.

Significant variation in these parameters should be regarded with suspicion, and may suggest the need for prompt re-sampling.

Medication Interfering with UDS

Medications can interfere with urine drug screens (Table **2**). It is important to check for these interactions when screens are positive. The confirmatory tests will identify a false positive.

Table 2. Selected false positives with UDS immunoassays.

Substance of Abuse	False Positives (Item ingested)	Comments
Opiates	Chlorpromazine, Dextromethorphan, Diphenhydramine, Fluorquinolones: Levofloxacin, Ciprofloxacin, Ofloxacin, Poppy Seeds, Quinine, Rifampin	Poppy seeds contain morphine Screens have limited sensitivity: positive for morphine could be codeine or heroin Very low ability to identify synthetic opioids
Methadone	Doxylamine (ex-high dose), Propoxyphene, Quetiapine, Verapamil	Expanded Opiate Test required for synthetics: fentanyl, hydrocodone, methadone, oxycodone, buprenorphine, tramadol

(Table 2) contd.....

Substance of Abuse	False Positives (Item ingested)	Comments
Amphetamines	Amantadine, Bupropion, Chlorpromazine, Desipramine, Epinephrine Fluoxetine, Labetalol, Methylphenidate, Phenylephrine, Phenylpropanolamine, Promethazine, Pseudoephedrine, Ranitidine, Trazodone, Trimethobenzamide, Vicks Vapor Spray MDMA, Ecstasy: methylenedioxy-methylamphetamine	Screen tests are highly cross reactive Very low specificity Not very diagnostic without confirmation No passive inhalation of methamphetamine will yield a positive test
Cocaine	Topical anesthetics with cocaine Coca-leaf Tea - illegal	Contains cocaine Tests for cocaine have high specificity to cocaine/ benzoylecgonine Very little cross reactivity
Cannabis	Dronabinol Efavirenz NSAIDS: Ibuprofen, Naproxen, Ketoprofen, Sulindac, Piroxicam; Pantoprazole (and other proton pump inhibitors) Surfactants in newborn body washes	Moderate specificity Marinol – prescription version Synthetic and natural THC differentiation requires special testing Passive inhalation would require patient participation in having it blown directly into the face in large amounts, unlikely to see with a cutoff of 50 ng/ml
Benzodiazepines	Oxaprozin, Sertraline	Test may not cover specific agents, will need to request
PCP	Chlorpromazine, Dextromethorphan, Diphenhydramine, Doxylamine, Ibuprofen, Imipramine, Ketamine, Meperidine, Thioridazine,Tramadol, Venlafaxine	
Buprenorphine	Amisulprde*, Sulpiride*	*not available in the US Buprenorphine cross reacts with morphine, codeine, dihydrocodeine

Adapted from references [1, 2, 4, 7]

SPECIAL CONSIDERATIONS

Opiate/Opioid Metabolism

Many UDS can be confounded by the presence of opioid/opiate metabolites (Fig. **1**). It is important to be aware of the metabolites of the medication being prescribed. Fentanyl has no metabolites and oxycodone does not metabolize into morphine so it is not detected by a routine UDS [3, 4].

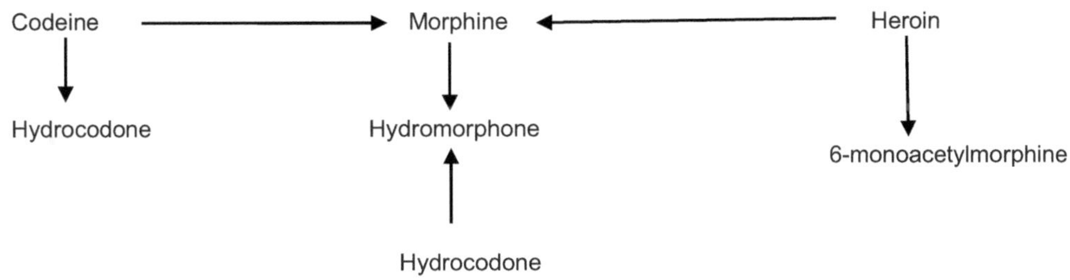

Fig. (1). Opiate/opioid metabolism.

Benzodiazepines

UDS tests for metabolites oxazepam and nordiazepam but not for all specific benzodiazepines. Not all benzodiazepines are associated with these metabolites including alprazolam and lorazepam. Depending on your laboratory you may be able to order a test of the specific agent.

Untested Substances

UDS is not able to detect some substances such as "bath salts", 3, 4-methylenedioxy-N-methyl amphetamine (MDMA), ketamine and methanol. An alternative test will be needed. Working with the laboratory doing the testing you can order tests for these and other substances of interest.

Altered Pharmacokinetic and Pharmacodynamic Parameters

Alterations in absorption (route of use), distribution, metabolism and elimination can affect the ability of the UDS to detect substances in the urine. For example, altering the pH of the urine to be more acidic can increase the elimination of methamphetamine.

SUMMARY

Urine drug screening can be a useful tool in the clinical setting. "Planned" random testing as part of a treatment agreement and contingency management can provide information on the success of the current plan. It can identify situations resulting in intense craving, personal and interpersonal issues that need to be addressed, and long-term withdrawal symptoms that need to be ameliorated. Consequences of a positive test on the patient's treatment should be clearly stated at the beginning of treatment. Urine samples need to be handled securely and any positive screens need to be verified with a confirmation test.

PATIENT INFORMATION SHEET – URINE DRUG SCREENS

What Role Does a Urine Drug Screen Play in the Treatment of a Substance Use Disorder?

A urine drug screen can be a motivating factor for you in maintaining your sobriety. It is a barometer of success and can indicate times that are hardest for you to stay off your substance. Illicit drug use may indicate issues such as interpersonal conflicts, stress, long-term withdrawal symptoms or craving that need to be addressed in treatment.

What Happens if my Urine Drug Screen is Positive?

Any positive urine screen should be confirmed by a more specific test. If this confirmation is positive, how that affects your treatment will depend on how the drug screen has been incorporated into your treatment plan.

Are there Medications that can Lead to a False Positive?

Yes, treatment with several medications can result in a false positive screen. If urine drug screening is part of your treatment plan you and your provider should review these medications frequently. If urine drug testing is a job requirement you need to know if any over-the-counter or prescription medications you use can cause false positives, ask your provider when new medications are added to your regimen.

I Heard that Poppy Seeds in Food can Lead to a Positive Test for Opiates. Is that True?

Yes, eating enough poppy seeds can lead to a false positive test. It will depend on the amount ingested and the level in the urine meeting the minimum threshold detected by a urine test.

Are there Ways to Neutralize Substances in the Urine to Hide Substance Use?

Many methods have been used in an attempt to fool a urine drug screen. However they don't work if urine samples are handled in a secure fashion in special urine collection cups that help detect efforts to confound testing.

If I am Around Someone Smoking Weed or Methamphetamine will that Cause my Urine to be Positive?

No. Breathing in someone else's "second hand smoke" will not cause a positive urine screen.

CONFLICT OF INTEREST

The author confirms that she has no conflict of interest to declare for this publication.

ACKNOWLEDGEMENTS

Declared none.

REFERENCES

[1] Markway EC, Baker SN. A review of the methods, interpretation, and limitations of the urine drug screen. Orthopedics 2011; 34(11): 877-81. [cited: 29th July 2013]. [http://dx.doi.org/10.3928/01477447-20110922-22] [PMID: 22050253]

[2] Cotten SW, Duncan DL, Burch EA, Seashore CJ, Hammett-Stabler CA. Unexpected interference of baby wash products with a cannabinoid (THC) immunoassay. Clin Biochem 2012; 45(9): 605-9. [http://dx.doi.org/10.1016/j.clinbiochem.2012.02.029] [PMID: 22465236]

[3] Manchikanti L, Atluri S, Trescot AM, Giordano J. Monitoring opioid adherence in chronic pain patients: tools, techniques, and utility. Pain Physician 2008; 11(2) (Suppl.): S155-80. [Opioids Special Issue]. [PMID: 18443638]

[4] Manchikanti L, Malla Y, Wargo BW, *et al.* Protocol for accuracy of point of care (POC) or in-office urine drug testing (immunoassay) in chronic pain patients: a prospective analysis of immunoassay and liquid chromatography tandem mass spectrometry (LC/MS/MS). Pain Physician 2010; 13(1): E1-E22. [PMID: 20119473]

[5] Standridge JB, Adams SM, Zotos AP. Urine drug screening: a valuable office procedure. Am Fam Physician 2010; 81(5): 635-40. [PMID: 20187600]

[6] Gourlay D, Heit HA, Caplan YH. Urine drug testing in clinical practice: dispelling the myths and designing strategies. California Academy of Family Physician. California: Academy of Family Physician 2006.

[7] Birch MA, Couchman L, Pietromartire S, *et al.* False-positive buprenorphine by CEDIA in patients prescribed amisulpride or sulpiride. J Anal Toxicol 2013; 37(4): 233-36. [http://dx.doi.org/10.1093/jat/bkt016]

CHAPTER 3

Genetics of Addiction

Imad Alsakaf[1,*] and **Subhash C. Bhatia**[2,3]

[1] *Creighton University School of Medicine, 3528 Dodge Street Omaha, NE 68131 USA*

[2] *Department of Psychiatry, Mental Health and Behavioral Sciences, Creighton University*

[3] *Department VA Nebraska- Western Iowa Health Care System 4101 Woolworth Ave Omaha, NE 68105, USA*

Abstract: Addictive disorders are complex diseases influenced by both genetic and environmental factors. Heritability of these disorders is moderate to high. Genes that increase the risk of addiction to a substance actually increase the risk of addiction to other substances. This means it is mainly through broad externalizing pathways that genes increase the risk of addiction. The current level of our knowledge in genetics is less than enough to have clinical applications. Probably, in the near future, we will be able to provide our patients with individualized report about their susceptibility to addiction.

Keywords: Environment, Genes, Genotype, Heritability, Phenotype, Risk, Susceptibility.

KEY LEARNING POINTS

1. Addictive disorders are complex diseases where genes, environment, stage of development and race play a part.
2. Based on twin studies heritability varies with the type of drug addiction.
3. Because of the co-occurrence of addictions and mental disorders it is possible that common genetic mechanisms play a part in both.

[*] **Corresponding author Imad Alsakaf:** Creighton University School of Medicine, 3528 Dodge Street Omaha, NE 68131 USA; Tel: 402-572-2483, Fax: 402-572-3472; Email: imad.alsakaf@alegent.org

4. Some specific genes have been identified *e.g.* for alcohol addiction protection, nicotine addiction.
5. Due to rapid advances in the field of genetics the answer to the association of genes and addiction is within our reach in the near future.

GENETICS OF ADDICTION

Both the environment and the genes contribute to degree of risk of developing these diseases.

The risk of heritability of addictive disorders is moderate to high and it is not the same among different substances. Moreover, factors like age, developmental stage, sex and race affect the degree of that risk [1].

Behaviors that are considered addictive are heterogeneous in their genetic origins and in their manifestations, which makes it more difficult to understand the heritability of these behaviors [1].

Twin studies help with quantifying the heritability of different addictive disorders. The heritability for nicotine dependence is 33-71% [2], alcohol dependence 48-66% [3], cannabis addiction 51-59% [4], cocaine use disorder 42-79% [5], opioid addiction 23% [6] and disordered gambling 49% [7]. Overall heritability for addiction to various substances of abuse is about 30% to 60% [1].

Twin studies suggest that specific genetic factors predispose some individuals to develop addictive disorders that co-occur with mental health disorders [1].

There is still a lot of a discussion about the use of the terms substance abuse, dependence and addiction. These terms are often used interchangeably.

Developing studies that help understand how genes influence addiction is difficult when the above terms are poorly delineated [1].

Recent publication of the DSM- 5 could have an impact on future studies, as the diagnosis of substance abuse and the diagnosis of substance dependence were removed from DSM-5 and replaced with the diagnoses of substance use disorder and non-substance use disorders or behavioral addictions, like gambling, have been added [8].

Researchers have discovered few specific genes that protect against or increase the risk of developing specific addictive disorders. For example, the (ALDH2) gene is protective against alcohol dependence because it decreases the ability of metabolizing acetaldehyde. The build up with acetaldehyde causes symptoms, like flushed face, anxiety, nausea and vomiting. This leads to decrease in alcohol use, which results in decreased risk of developing alcohol dependence [9].

Gene cluster CHRNA5/A3/B4, which is found on chromosome 15 is amongst the most replicated for association with nicotine addiction [10]. Interestingly, this gene cluster on chromosome 15 is also associated with cocaine addiction. No consistent association has been reported for cannabinoid receptor 1 gene. The gene encoding the mu-opiod receptor OPRM1 has been extensively studied as to its role in opioid addiction but this relationship has not been consistently replicated. For disordered gambling dopamine 1 receptor encoding gene (DRD1) was reported to be associated with this disorder but a recent study did not support this association [11].

Some of the most important genes for substance addiction are the dopaminergic genes, especially the D2 receptor genes, mainly because of the important role of dopamine in the reward system [1].

While providing education to patients, we need to avoid conveying the idea that alcohol dependence is genetic as we know that a significant portion of the risk is actually environmental [1].

SUMMARY

Addictive disorders have genetic basis with heritability risk ranging from 23 to 79%. A few susceptibility and protective genes have been identified.

PATIENT EDUCATION SHEET

What is the Relationship of Genes and Addictions?

Addictions are complex diseases like diabetes. Genes, age, sex, development stage and environment play a role in the development of addiction.

Is this Genetic Transmission for Addictions Dominant?

Addictions are not autosomal dominant but recessive with variable penetrance and expressivity between generations.

Do We have Gene Therapies for Addictions?

Not at present.

Where can I Get More Information?

www.drugabuse.gov or information@nida.nih.gov

CONFLICT OF INTEREST

The authors confirm that they have no conflict of interest to declare for this publication.

ACKNOWLEDGEMENTS

Declared none.

REFERENCES

[1] Edwards AC, Svikis DS, Pickens RW, Dick DM. Genetic influences on addiction. Prim Psychiatry 2009; 16(8): 40-6.

[2] Edwards AC, Maes HH, Pedersen NL, Kendler KS. A population-based twin study of the genetic and environmental relationship of major depression, regular tobacco use and nicotine dependence. Psychol Med 2011; 41(2): 395-405. [http://dx.doi.org/10.1017/S0033291710000589] [PMID: 20406522]

[3] Heath AC, Whitfield JB, Madden PA, *et al.* Towards a molecular epidemiology of alcohol dependence: analysing the interplay of genetic and environmental risk factors. Br J Psychiatry Suppl 2001; 40: s33-40. [http://dx.doi.org/10.1192/bjp.178.40.s33] [PMID: 11315223]

[4] Verweij KJ, Zietsch BP, Lynskey MT, *et al.* Genetic and environmental influences on cannabis use initiation and problematic use: a meta-analysis of twin studies. Addiction 2010; 105(3): 417-30. [http://dx.doi.org/10.1111/j.1360-0443.2009.02831.x] [PMID: 20402985]

[5] van den Bree MB, Johnson EO, Neale MC, Pickens RW. Genetic and environmental influences on drug use and abuse/dependence in male and female twins. Drug Alcohol Depend 1998; 52(3): 231-41.

[http://dx.doi.org/10.1016/S0376-8716(98)00101-X] [PMID: 9839149]

[6] Kendler KS, Karkowski LM, Neale MC, Prescott CA. Illicit psychoactive substance use, heavy use, abuse, and dependence in a US population-based sample of male twins. Arch Gen Psychiatry 2000; 57(3): 261-9.
[http://dx.doi.org/10.1001/archpsyc.57.3.261] [PMID: 10711912]

[7] Slutske WS, Zhu G, Meier MH, Martin NG. Genetic and environmental influences on disordered gambling in men and women. Arch Gen Psychiatry 2010; 67(6): 624-30.
[http://dx.doi.org/10.1001/archgenpsychiatry.2010.51] [PMID: 20530012]

[8] Diagnostic and Statistical Manual of Mental Disorders. 5th ed., Arlington, VA: American Psychiatric Association 2013.

[9] Luo X, Kranzler HR, Zuo L, Wang S, Schork NJ, Gelernter J. Diplotype trend regression analysis of the ADH gene cluster and the ALDH2 gene: multiple significant associations with alcohol dependence. Am J Hum Genet 2006; 78(6): 973-87.
[http://dx.doi.org/10.1086/504113] [PMID: 16685648]

[10] Keskitalo-Vuokko K, Pitkäniemi J, Broms U, *et al.* Associations of nicotine intake measures with CHRN genes in Finnish smokers. Nicotine Tob Res 2011; 13(8): 686-90.
[http://dx.doi.org/10.1093/ntr/ntr059] [PMID: 21498873]

[11] Lobo DS, Souza RP, Tong RP, *et al.* Association of functional variants in the dopamine D2-like receptors with risk for gambling behaviour in healthy Caucasian subjects. Biol Psychol 2010; 85(1): 33-7.
[http://dx.doi.org/10.1016/j.biopsycho.2010.04.008] [PMID: 20452395]

CHAPTER 4

Dual Diagnosis

R. Dario Pulido*

Mental Health and Behavioral Sciences, Department VA Nebraska-Western Iowa Health Care System, 4101 Woolworth Ave. Omaha, NE 68105, USA

Abstract: Dual diagnosis exists when there is a substance use disorder occurring in conjunction with another non-substance mental health diagnosis. The presence of dual diagnosis is common and poses significant challenges to health care providers, due to both the increased severity and poorer treatment outcomes compared to when there is a single condition. Substance use disorders may develop in response to a mental health condition, although this is not always the case. A key diagnostic task is to conduct a thorough assessment that considers a full range of issues. Treatment should attempt to address both aspects of a dual diagnosis in an integrated and coordinated manner. If this is not possible, treatment for both conditions should at least be concurrent. This is in contrast to past perspectives embracing a sequential approach. Treatments for dual diagnoses are effective and may include a variety of interventions including psychotherapy, pharmacotherapy, and community self-help groups. The current chapter utilizes a case example to illustrate many of the relevant issues.

Keywords: Assessment, Comorbid conditions, Comorbidity, Dual diagnoses, Dual diagnosis, Substance use disorder, Treatment.

KEY LEARNING POINTS

1. Dual diagnoses occur when a person suffers from both a substance use disorder and another mental health diagnosis.
2. Dual diagnoses are very common.
3. A thorough assessment is crucial to identify comorbid disorders.

* **Corresponding author R. Dario Pulido:** Mental Health and Behavioral Sciences, Department VA Nebraska-Western Iowa Health Care System, 4101 Woolworth Ave. Omaha, NE 68105, USA; Tel: (402) 995-4301; Fax (402) 995-3277; Email: ruben.pulido@va.gov

Subhash C. Bhatia (Ed.)

4. Treatment options include pharmacotherapy, psychotherapy, and use of community supports (*e.g.* 12-step groups).
5. Treatment should target both conditions in a concurrent or integrated manner.

CLINICAL VIGNETTE

Ms. Q is a 34-year-old Caucasian woman who presents to your clinic complaining of sleep problems and feeling "overwhelmed". She states that her mood has been "down" for nearly a year since about the time of her separation from her fiancé with whom she lived. She has had significant difficulty maintaining contacts with friends and family and has little motivation to engage in activities she used to enjoy. She has grown increasingly isolated and her work is suffering due to problems with attendance and concentration.

An inquiry into current substance use patterns reveals daily alcohol use. She drinks approximately 4-6 shots of vodka most nights, which she says helps her sleep. She notes increasing tolerance over time and several failed efforts to quit. More recently, she has found herself taking a drink in the morning "to avoid the shakes". She began drinking heavily near the end of her last relationship and has continued to drink despite being charged with a DUI.

Further discussion reveals a significant preoccupation with safety and beliefs about the world being "totally dangerous." She reports walking in her neighborhood only when accompanied by her large dog and repeatedly patrolling her house with the dog at her side to ensure that all doors and windows are locked. Sleep is a significant problem for Ms. Q, and she states that she cannot easily fall asleep unless she is intoxicated. Even when intoxicated she is only able to sleep for 4-5 hours per night, partly because she is plagued by nightmares. The content of the nightmares is related to episodes of domestic violence that occurred during her relationship. The worst episode involved her partner brandishing a knife and threatening to slash Ms. Q's throat. This event was terrifying and eventually led to Ms. Q's flight from the relationship. Images of the violent episodes (particularly the threats at knifepoint) frequently intrude into her consciousness and cause emotional and physical agitation. She currently feels jumpy and easily irritated. She also reports having a sense that her future will somehow be cut short. She has never told anyone about the abuse and she makes significant efforts to avoid reminders of the relationship.

BACKGROUND

The term dual diagnosis is defined in this chapter as the presence of a substance use disorder (of a substance other than nicotine and caffeine) in conjunction with at least one other non-substance mental health diagnosis. Mental health issues commonly seen in dual diagnoses include mood disorders, such as major depressive disorder and bipolar disorders, anxiety or trauma- and stressor-related disorders including posttraumatic stress disorder (PTSD), and psychotic illnesses such as schizophrenia. A broad definition of dual diagnosis is used in the current chapter rather than the more restrictive definition requiring the presence of a severe and persistent mental illness (*e.g.* bipolar or psychotic disorder). The term dual diagnosis as used in this chapter also excludes the presence of multiple mental health conditions without an associated substance use problem.

The presence of dual diagnoses poses a significant challenge to healthcare providers. Patients with dual diagnoses may not respond as well to mental health treatment, experience higher relapse rates, and have poorer treatment compliance. Additionally, symptoms in this population may be more severe than for those with just one condition [10, 11]. These factors, in addition to others such as likely increased functional impairments make caring for the dually diagnosed more complex.

Dual diagnoses are common. Large epidemiological studies such as the National Comorbidity Study, have found that over 40% of those who were diagnosed with a substance use disorder in the past 12 months also had another non-substance mental health disorder during the same time period. Lifetime comorbidities are even greater, with rates of 41-65% of those who have had a substance use disorder also having had a mental health problem at some point in their lives [8]. The disorders with the greatest likelihoods of lifetime prevalence in conjunction with alcohol use problems are conduct disorder and antisocial personality disorder, followed by anxiety and affective disorders [7]. More recent large-scale studies confirm the high incidence of current and lifetime comorbidity for substance use disorders and mental health issues [3, 5, 6].

Although not invariable, some general patterns do emerge regarding the trajectories of comorbid disorders. Notably, for those individuals with a history of both alcohol misuse and another mental health problem, the mental disorder more frequently predates the alcohol problem. This does not hold true, however in the case of co-occurring alcohol and mood disorders among men. For that population, substance use more frequently emerges prior to the mood disorder [8].

As suggested in the vignette, in some instances substance use may develop, in part, as an effort to manage a mental health condition. In the case of Ms. Q, alcohol use may have developed as a means to manage symptoms of PTSD. Clinical experience reveals that alcohol use at times might decrease anxiety, reduce initial insomnia and reduce the recall of nightmares in those with PTSD (especially for those who drink to "black out"). Paradoxically however, when patients use alcohol to manage PTSD symptoms, the symptoms often return with greater intensity during alcohol withdrawal. This in turn may foster further drinking to reduce the felt agitation, leading to a pernicious cycle of PTSD and alcohol use [4]. For some individuals with PTSD, the effort may be to avoid sleep (and nightmares) altogether by staying up through the use of amphetamines or cocaine.

Being that primary care providers are often the patient's initial point of contact with the health care system, these providers play a crucial role in identifying problems and helping patients access relevant services. Many patients may not recognize a need for treatment or have knowledge of the types of services that are available. Input and direction from primary care providers is invaluable in helping patients address their difficulties and achieve a state of better emotional and physical health.

DIAGNOSTIC CONSIDERATIONS

A key diagnostic challenge in dealing with individuals suffering from comorbid conditions is obtaining a complete diagnostic picture. Both patient and clinician factors may hinder a clinician's pursuit of this objective. Patients may experience different levels of stigma regarding comorbid conditions. For example, a patient may find it more acceptable to have a "drinking problem" rather than be diagnosed with depression. As a result, the patient may be inclined to reveal information about one set of difficulties but obfuscate the other. On the other hand, providers may have a tendency to identify one psychiatric issue and neglect to search for other conditions. For example, a provider might attribute struggles with mood or motivation solely to a patient's known substance use and fail to identify a comorbid depressive disorder. In the case of Ms. Q, the provider may have simply focused on alcohol use, thereby missing a significant level of trauma-related symptoms.

Another important issue in the diagnosis of comorbid conditions, is that other mental health problems may occur as a consequence of substance intoxication or withdrawal (substance-induced). These problems may be transitory, and can often resolve simply with a period of sobriety. However, if the other mental health conditions are known to predate the substance use, or if the conditions persist to a significant extent after drug and/or alcohol use is discontinued, one should consider an independent diagnosis other than substance-induced [1].

In the case of Ms. Q, no mood or substance use problems were present prior to her experiences of mistreatment at the hands of her partner. She reports that symptoms including fearfulness, sleep problems, and intrusive imagery developed following her traumatic experience. She also described her alcohol use as a means to help her feel calm enough to deal with her ex-fiancé's past abusive and unpredictable behavior, and as a coping strategy to deal with intrusive recollections including nightmares. Ms. Q's symptoms are consistent with Posttraumatic Stress Disorder (PTSD). Additionally, her symptoms meet criteria for a diagnosis of Alcohol Use Disorder, Moderate. In conjunction with these syndromes, she has grown increasingly depressed, although affective symptoms do not fully satisfy the diagnostic criteria for major depressive disorder and appear to be secondary to PTSD and alcohol use.

It is also important for the primary care provider to assess the degree of functional impairment present. Functioning may be assessed in relation to a variety of domains including work, self-care, recreation, interpersonal relationships, and neurocognitive status. Inquiry about how the patient is doing in each of these areas can yield important data to be used in determining the best course of treatment. In the case of Ms. Q, functioning was significantly impaired. Her work suffered due to hangovers, concentration problems that made it difficult to complete tasks, and attendance problems related to anxiety about being around others. Ms. Q also suffered significant problems in the areas of recreation and socialization. She found herself no longer exercising or spending time with friends. She became estranged from others and often avoided calls from friends and family. Neurocognitively, Ms. Q. reported ongoing problems with concentration and focus, often finding it hard to complete work assignments, watch TV, or even read the newspaper.

TREATMENT CONSIDERATIONS

As in any clinical situation, treatment priorities must first focus on the immediate health and safety of the individual. Providers should follow available treatment guidelines regarding urgent health and safety issues, including protocols for detoxification and management of withdrawal. In this case, Ms. Q did not require a medically supervised detoxification.

Previous perspectives on treatment for the dually diagnosed endorsed a sequential approach in which providers were encouraged to identify a "primary" diagnosis to treat first, and then after that has been adequately managed, provide services for the "secondary" condition. Current clinical evidence, however, strongly supports the idea of integrated treatment of comorbid conditions [9 - 11]. At a minimum, treatment should involve the concurrent provision of services for substance use and mental health issues. Ideally, there should be a high degree of coordination between the treatment programs or providers.

Although difficulties associated with dual diagnosis may be more intense or complex than in single disorder cases, treatments are effective. A recent review of treatment studies shows that existing treatments for psychiatric issues and for substance use are both effective in helping those with dual diagnoses. In other words, treatments that work for the singly diagnosed also work for the dually diagnosed [12].

Treatment for dual diagnoses may include a variety of interventions including pharmacotherapy, psychotherapy, and participation in community self-help groups. In the current case, as the primary care provider had experience with relevant pharmacotherapy, Ms. Q was prescribed medications for PTSD symptoms. The most common first line treatment for both anxiety and depressive disorders are the selective serotonin reuptake inhibitors (SSRIs). In complex cases, a provider may wish to refer the patient to a psychiatrist for psychotropic medication management.

In addition to psychopharmacological interventions, the provider referred Ms. Q to a psychotherapist who provided Cognitive Behavior Therapy (CBT) for PTSD and depressive symptoms. Work with the therapist also supported Ms. Q's sobriety in relation to alcohol. It is strongly recommended that referrals be made to psychotherapists who have experience and specialized training in dealing with the relevant issues. Finally, her primary care provider also recommended that Ms. Q attend Alcoholics Anonymous for further support.

Although Alcoholics Anonymous is the largest and most well known of the 12-step groups, many different specialized groups following a 12-step model are available. These include Narcotics Anonymous, Cocaine Anonymous, and other groups related to compulsive behaviors such as Gambler's Anonymous, and Sex and Love Addicts Anonymous. Listings of local groups and meeting times can be easily accessed *via* the internet.

If a patient is not interested in a 12-step approach due to its spiritual nature, other community supports are available that do not use a spiritual orientation, such as Agnostics Anonymous, Rational Recovery, and Smart Recovery. If the patient is not interested in abstinence as a goal, a harm reduction approach may be used within the context of psychotherapy with the aim of reducing substance use to manageable levels that have minimal negative consequences.

World Health Organization guidelines around alcohol use suggest that for contained or limited use (*i.e.* harm reduction), contraindications include prior substance use disorders, morning shaking, history of unsuccessful attempts to cut down, serious mental illness, hypertension, pregnancy, liver disease, and taking medications that react with alcohol [2]. Although, these guidelines are for alcohol, parallels may be drawn for other substances.

In addition to outpatient treatment, as described in this case example, inpatient treatment may also be appropriate. Typical options include a brief detoxification period, a short-term substance use treatment stay (usually about a month), or an admission to a psychiatric unit if there are concerns about safety (*e.g.* suicide). In some instances, longer-term and more comprehensive residential treatment options may be available.

TREATMENT OUTCOMES

Ms. Q was relieved to hear that her difficulties were related to known and common conditions, and were not a sign of her "going crazy." Having the diagnosis of PTSD as a way to understand her problems provided her with some reassurance, as did knowing there are effective treatments. Ms. Q also recognized that her alcohol use was problematic. However, she was able to resist excessive self-blame and criticism by realizing that her drinking, at least initially, was an effort to cope with her PTSD symptoms.

Ms. Q agreed to treatment with an antidepressant medication, which relieved some agitation and improved her mood. She also began seeing a psychotherapist and eventually participated in Cognitive Processing Therapy, a cognitive-behavioral treatment for PTSD. In time, and with ongoing psychotherapy, Ms. Q's PTSD symptoms were significantly diminished. Although she still struggled with concerns about safety and periodically thought about her abuse, she no longer met full criteria for this diagnosis. With the PTSD better managed, she felt less of a need to utilize alcohol to help her deal with those symptoms and was able to maintain sobriety with the support of regular AA attendance.

Overall, Ms. Q's case had a very favorable outcome. PTSD symptoms were reduced to the point that they no longer satisfied criteria for a diagnosis of PTSD. Abstinence from alcohol was eventually achieved. Overall functioning improved to the point that she was able to work effectively and socialize without significant anxiety. She was able to re-establish important connections with friends and family.

SUMMARY

Dual diagnosis refers to the presence of a substance use disorder in conjunction with at least one other non-substance mental health diagnosis. Dual diagnosis is a significant and common problem, which poses particular challenges in evaluation and treatment. A careful and thorough assessment is necessary for accurate diagnosis. Existing treatments are effective for this population and should be provided in a concurrent and coordinated manner.

DUAL DIAGNOSIS - PATIENT INFORMATION SHEET

What is a Dual Diagnosis?

"Dual Diagnosis" is the presence of a substance use disorder (of a substance other than nicotine or caffeine) in conjunction with at least one other non-substance mental health diagnosis.

How is it Treated?

Treatment may include medications, psychotherapy, and/or use of community supports (*e.g.* AA). It is encouraged that you engage in treatment for both conditions as soon as possible and at the same time.

What can I Expect in Psychotherapy?

You can expect to have regularly scheduled appointments with a trained professional who will develop a treatment plan with you to address key problems associated with mental health and/or substance use. In most circumstances treatment is confidential. Sessions will involve talking about your difficulties in certain ways aimed at relieving distressing symptoms and/or reducing substance use.

What are the Long-term Outcomes?

Outcomes are favorable if you utilize support services and actively engage in treatment/recovery activities.

What are Some "Do's and Don'ts" Related to Having a Dual Diagnosis?

- Don't use and drive
- Do maintain a daily structure
- Do have sober friends
- Do attend support groups
- Do access mental health treatment

What are Some Available Resources?

- American Psychiatric Association: www.healthyminds.org
- American Psychological Association: www.apahelpcenter.org
- Mental Health America: www.nmha.org
- National Alliance on Mental Illness: www.nami.org
- National Institute of Mental health: www.nimh.nih.gov
- National Institute on Drug Abuse: www.nida.nih.gov

What should I do Next if I Think I have a Problem?

Reach out. Talk with loved ones, trusted friends, or medical providers. Use the available resources (above) and consider professional help. Remember that you have options and do not have to continue suffering in this way.

CONFLICT OF INTEREST

The author confirms that he has no conflict of interest to declare for this publication.

ACKNOWLEDGEMENTS

Declared none.

REFERENCES

[1] Diagnostic and Statistical Manual of Mental Disorders. 5th ed., Arlington, VA: American Psychiatric Association 2013.

[2] Babor TF, Higgins-Biddle JC. Brief intervention for hazardous and harmful drinking: A manual for use in primary care. World Health Organization, Department of Mental Health and Substance Dependence. Available from: http://whqlibdoc.who.int/hq/2001/WHO_MSD_MSB_01.6b.pdf 2001.

[3] Grant BF, Stinson FS, Dawson DA, *et al.* Prevalence and co-occurrence of substance use disorders and independent mood and anxiety disorders: results from the National Epidemiologic Survey on Alcohol and Related Conditions. Arch Gen Psychiatry 2004; 61(8): 807-16. [http://dx.doi.org/10.1001/archpsyc.61.8.807] [PMID: 15289279]

[4] Jacobsen LK, Southwick SM, Kosten TR. Substance use disorders in patients with posttraumatic stress disorder: a review of the literature. Am J Psychiatry 2001; 158(8): 1184-90. [http://dx.doi.org/10.1176/appi.ajp.158.8.1184] [PMID: 11481147]

[5] Kessler RC, Berglund P, Demler O, Jin R, Merikangas KR, Walters EE. Lifetime prevalence and age-of-onset distributions of DSM-IV disorders in the National Comorbidity Survey Replication. Arch Gen Psychiatry 2005; 62(6): 593-602. [http://dx.doi.org/10.1001/archpsyc.62.6.593] [PMID: 15939837]

[6] Kessler RC, Chiu WT, Demler O, Merikangas KR, Walters EE. Prevalence, severity, and comorbidity of 12-month DSM-IV disorders in the National Comorbidity Survey Replication. Arch Gen Psychiatry 2005; 62(6): 617-27. [http://dx.doi.org/10.1001/archpsyc.62.6.617] [PMID: 15939839]

[7] Kessler RC, Crum RM, Warner LA, Nelson CB, Schulenberg J, Anthony JC. Lifetime co-occurrence of DSM-III-R alcohol abuse and dependence with other psychiatric disorders in the National Comorbidity Survey. Arch Gen Psychiatry 1997; 54(4): 313-21. [http://dx.doi.org/10.1001/archpsyc.1997.01830160031005] [PMID: 9107147]

[8] Kessler RC, Nelson CB, McGonagle KA, Edlund MJ, Frank RG, Leaf PJ. The epidemiology of co-occurring addictive and mental disorders: implications for prevention and service utilization. Am J Orthopsychiatry 1996; 66(1): 17-31. [http://dx.doi.org/10.1037/h0080151] [PMID: 8720638]

[9] Mueser KT, Drake RE, Miles K. The course and treatment of substance use disorder in persons with severe mental illness. Treatment of Drug-dependent Individuals with Comorbid Disorders. Nida Res Monogr. 1997; 172: pp. 86-109.

[10] Mueser KT, Noordsy DL, Drake RE, Fox L. Integrated treatment for dual disorders. NY: Guilford Press 2003.

[11] Sheehan MF. Dual diagnosis. Psychiatr Q 1993; 64(2): 107-34. [http://dx.doi.org/10.1007/BF01065865] [PMID: 8316597]

[12] Tiet QQ, Mausbach B. Treatments for patients with dual diagnosis: a review. Alcohol Clin Exp Res 2007; 31(4): 513-36. [PMID: 17374031]

CHAPTER 5

Pharmacologic Treatment for Psychiatric Disorders Associated with Substance Use Disorders: An Overview

Teri Gabel*

VA Nebraska Western Iowa Health Care System, Clinical Pharmacy Specialist - Mental Health, Omaha, NE 68105; Department of Psychiatry, University Of Nebraska College of Medicine Omaha NE 68198; Drug Therapy Consultants, PC 5116 N 116 St, Omaha NE 68164 USA

Abstract: Management of substance use disorders is challenging, there are no medications that directly treat the use disorders, substitution therapy in opioid use disorders and potential anti-craving medications for alcohol use disorder are the closest available. Successful management of withdrawal syndromes and craving can improve the chances of sobriety. The presence of underlying medical and psychiatric disorders can derail attempts at long term sobriety if not managed. This chapter provides information on medications commonly used in the management of withdrawal symptoms and co-morbid psychiatric disorders, such as depression and anxiety, in the dually diagnosed patient. Tables of medications from the following classes are included: benzodiazepines and other antianxiety agents, antidepressants, mood stabilizers, anticonvulsants and antipsychotic medications. Key points in the patient specific selection, dosing and monitoring of these medications and management of their side effects are identified. Insomnia can derail sobriety and needs to be addressed. Information on sleep hygiene and medications for insomnia are also presented. Information on the individualization of treatment is also discussed. It is important to note that many of the medications presented in this chapter are being used for both US FDA labeled and off-label indications.

* **Corresponding author Teri Gabel:** VA Nebraska Western Iowa Health Care System, Clinical Pharmacy Specialist - Mental Health, Omaha, NE 68105; Department of Psychiatry, University Of Nebraska College of Medicine Omaha NE 68198; Drug Therapy Consultants, PC 5116 N 116 St, Omaha NE 68164 USA; Tel: (402) 493-5222; Email: pharmdherb@gmail.com

Subhash C. Bhatia (Ed.)

Keywords: Anticonvulsants, Antidepressants, Antipsychotic, Anxiety, Benzodiazepines, Depression, Insomnia, Mood stabilizers, Psychotic symptoms.

KEY LEARNING POINTS

1. Co-morbid psychiatric and medical diagnoses need to be adequately treated.
2. Medications do not treat substance use disorders but manage associated symptoms.
3. Effectively managing the symptoms of withdrawal and craving can improve outcomes.
4. Medication choice must be carefully matched to the individual.
5. Many medications are used off-label in the management of substance use disorders and their symptoms.

INTRODUCTION

In the management of substance use disorders, pharmacologic interventions are generally used for symptomatic treatment of withdrawal and intoxication states or the management of underlying or co-morbid psychiatric diagnoses. Very few substance use disorders have FDA approved medications that can be used to decrease craving and/or assist with sobriety, the exception is opioid abuse, which has substitution therapies that are FDA approved [1]. Therefore, many medications listed below are used off-label in an attempt to assist the patient in their relapsing and remitting battle with substance use or managing symptoms due to anxiety, mood, psychotic or sleep disorders.

Benzodiazepines (Table 1)

Targets: intoxication, withdrawal states, agitation

- Ongoing use of benzodiazepines in patients with substance use disorders should be avoided if possible. In situations of acute intoxication or withdrawal the use of benzodiazepines may be indicated for a short period of time.
- For acute use, lorazepam is generally the medication of choice. In some situations, a longer acting agent such as clonazepam, chlordiazepoxide or diazepam may be indicated. Choice is determined by reason for use, the required route of administration and the presence of active metabolites resulting in a

longer duration of action.

Table 1. Selected benzodiazepines.

Agent	Equivalent Dose*	Pharmacokinetics/Pharmacology	Dosing Routes Available
Chlordiazepoxide	25mg	Onset: Slow (45-60 min) Half-life: 24-96+ hours 4-5 active metabolites	Oral IM: absorption is erratic and use is not recommended
Clonazepam	0.5mg	Onset: Intermediate (30 min) Half-life: 24 hours Insignificant active metabolites	Oral
Diazepam	5mg	Onset: Rapid (15 min) Half-life: 20-89+ hours 2-3 Active metabolites	Oral IV (max rate 5mg/minute) IM: absorption is adequate in the deltoid only
Lorazepam	1mg	Onset: Intermediate (30 min) Half-life: 12 hours NO active metabolites	Oral IV (max rate 2mg/minute) IM: good absorption anywhere

*Monitor the patient, conflicting data exists here. Adapted from references [2, 3]

Antidepressants

Targets: Depression, Anxiety, Impulsivity

- Medication selection will depend on patient and medication variables. Patients with preexisting depression and/or anxiety should continue to be treated during treatment for addictive disorders. Depression and anxiety can also develop during treatment and as a side effect of medications such as naltrexone and acamprosate, and needs to be addressed.
- All antidepressants carry a Black Box Warning regarding new onset suicidal ideation and behavior in children, adolescents, and young adults (<25yrs). Use of antidepressants must balance risk *versus* benefit.
- The Selective Serotonin Re-uptake Inhibitors (SSRI) and the Serotonin and Norepinephrine Reuptake Inhibitors (SNRIs) are used in the treatment of both depression and anxiety with good effectiveness and safety profiles and generic versions are available.
- Mirtazapine an agent with a different mechanism of action, alpha-2 auto-receptor blockade which results in elevated levels of serotonin and

norepinephrine, is also effective in the treatment of depression and of anxiety (off-label use).

- Bupropion blocks the reuptake of norepinephrine and dopamine and is effective in depression. It may be helpful with, or may worsen anxiety, and is used in smoking cessation.
- In the treatment of pain syndromes, the judicious use of tricyclic antidepressants (TCAs) and SNRIs may be of benefit in the management of depression, anxiety and pain.
- Use of antidepressant agents in patients with a personal or family history of bipolar disorder can result in the induction of a manic episode. Close monitoring is recommended and use combined with a mood stabilizer may be necessary.

Serotonin Syndrome

Presumed pathophysiology: activation of the 5HT-1A receptors in brainstem and spinal cord neurons resulting in enhanced serotonin transmission. Fatality results primarily when it goes unrecognized.

Onset: 3 - 4 days, Duration: Usually self-limiting, typically resolves 24 hours after discontinuing offending agents.

Syndrome Presentation

Changes in mental status, confusion, hypomania, hyperreflexia, myoclonus, diaphoresis, shivering, tremor, diarrhea, incoordination.

Treatment

1. Discontinue the offending agents.
2. Monitor/Supportive Care: Assist with respiration if required.
3. Medications: (possibly helpful)
   Cyproheptadine 4mg PO Q 1 hr x 3-4 doses.
   Methylsergide: 2mg PO Q 6 hr x 3-4 doses.
   Others as needed for agitation, seizures, hypertension and hyperthermia.

SSRI Withdrawal Phenomenon

Very similar to serotonin syndrome but less severe, more common with short half-life agents on abrupt discontinuation.

- Taper SSRIs slowly if symptoms become severe go back up to a dose that relieves them and then taper slowly.
- Fluoxetine has a very long half-life and may not require tapering. If symptoms occur, restart medication and taper as tolerated.

Table 2. Selected antidepressant agents.

Medication	Dosing Guidelines	Kinetics and Pharmacology	Side Effects
Serotonin Reuptake Inhibitors			
Fluoxetine (Prozac)	Initial dose: 10 - 20 mg a day Average dose: 20-80mg daily	Half-life: 7 days on average Fluoxetine + norfluoxetine (active metabolite) Inhibits CYP 2D6 > 3A4 May affect QTc	**Side effects**: *Non-selective* activation of serotonin receptors Serotonin Receptor Stimulation **5HT1A:** Antidepressant, Antianxiety, Anti-bulimia, Anti-obsessive-compulsive **5HT1D:** Anti-migraine **5HT2:** Causes Anxiety, Akathisia, Agitation, Insomnia, Panic attacks, Sexual Dysfunction **5HT3:** Causes Nausea, GI distress, Diarrhea, Headache *Blockade at these receptors antagonizes these actions *Most stimulating*: Prozac > Lexapro > Zoloft > Celexa > Paxil > Luvox *Most diarrhea*: Zolft > Paxil > Prozac > Celexa ≥ Lexapro > Luvox All cause photosensitivity Hyponatremia – all can cause Panic disorder – start with lower doses OCD will require higher doses
Sertraline (Zoloft)	Initial dose:25mg a day Average daily dose: 150-200mg	Half-life: 24 hours Few drug interactions Little effect on QTc	
Paroxetine (Paxil)	Initial dose: 10 - 20 mg a day Maintenance for depression: 40-60mg for OCD higher	Half-life: 24 hours No active metabolite Inhibits CYP 2D6 May affect QTc	
Citalopram (Celexa)	Initial dose: 10-20 mg a day Average daily doses: Adult: 20-40mg* (≤ 60yr) Geri (> 60yr): max 20mg/day* *Max dose per FDA due to concerns of QTc prolongation	Half-life: 24 hours Metabolites less active than parent compound Slight Inhibition of CYP 1A2, 2D6, 2C19 Substrate for 3A4 (parent) and 2C19 (metabolism) May affect QTc in higher doses	
Escitalopram (Lexapro)	10-20mg daily	Half-life: 24 hours Few drug interactions Little effect on QTc	

(Table 2) contd.....

Medication	Dosing Guidelines	Kinetics and Pharmacology	Side Effects
SSRI + 5HT1 partial agonism			
Vilazodone (Viibryd)	Start: 10mg /day with food x 7 days Increase to 20mg /day with food x 7 days then to 40mg/day with food Max Dose: 80mg/day No dose adjustment required for Geriatric patients	Half-life: 24 hours Use lower doses if in combination with CYP3A4 inhibitors, 3A4 inducers will decrease vilazodone levels Vilazodone may inhibit CYP 2C8 No QTc prolongation to 80mg/day	Diarrhea, nausea, vomiting, insomnia Food enhances absorption

5HT = Serotonin; CYP= Cytochrome P450; QTc= Corrected QT interval on EKG; OCD= Obsessive Compulsive Disorder. (Adapted from references [2 - 4]).

Table 3. Other antidepressants.

Dual Acting Agents: Increase Serotonin and Norepinephrine			
Venlafaxine (Effexor)	Initial dose: 25mg BID Range: 225-350mg Max:375mg/d SA allows for once daily dosing.	Half-life: 12 hours No Inhibition Active metabolite,O-D-venlafaxine	Stimulates all serotonin receptors Noradrenergic stimulation, DA side effects possible but uncommon, Photosensitivity Dose dependent hypertension (> 375mg/day) very patient variable
Duloxetine (Cymbalta)	Initial dose: 20mg BID Range: 40-60mg/day Max: 60mg/day Higher doses for pain	Half-life: 12 hours Active metabolites CPY 2D6,1A2 Inhibits CYP 2D6	Stimulation, insomnia, nausea, GI upset, constipation/diarrhea, dizziness, anorexia Sexual dysfunction men >>> women
Mirtazapine (Remeron)	Initial dose: 15mg Range: 30-45 Max: 60mg	Half-life: 24hours No inhibition	Fewer GI side effects Sedation and weight gain most common, At higher doses may be more stimulating, decreased weight gain Photosensitivity Little to no sexual dysfunction
Tricyclic Antidepressants (dual agents)			

(Table 3) contd.....

<table>
<tr><td>Amitriptyline
(Elavil)</td><td>Initial Dosing: 25 - 50 mg HS
Range: 150-200mg/day
*Chronic pain: 25 -100mg / day
*Primary use</td><td>Half-life: 24 hours
Metabolized via CYP 1A2 and CPY 2D6
active metabolite: nortryptiline
Blood Level: > 100 ng/ml (amit+nort)</td><td rowspan="3">Common Side Effects:
Antihistaminergic*
Anticholinergic**
Antiadrenergic***

Photosensitivity
Sexual Dysfunction
Syndrome of Inappropriate of Anti Diuretic Hormone (SIADH) secretion

Side effects same as above for nortryptiline and desipramine but less severe

Nortryptiline: least orthostatic
Desipramine: least anticholinergic and least weight gain</td></tr>
<tr><td>Nortryptiline
(Pamelor)</td><td>Initial dose: 25 - 50 mg
Range: 100-125mg/day</td><td>Half-life: 24 hours
Metabolized via CPY 2D6
Blood Level: 50-150 ng/ml
Twice as potent as other TCAs</td></tr>
<tr><td>Desipramine
(Norpramin)</td><td>Initial dose: 25 - 50 mg HS
Range: 150-200mg/day</td><td>Half-life: 24 hours
Metabolized via 2D6
Blood Level: > 100 ng/ml</td></tr>
<tr><td colspan="4">Increased Levels of Norepinephrine and Dopamine</td></tr>
<tr><td>Bupropion
(Wellbutrin, Zyban)</td><td>Initial dose: 75mg BID
Maintenance:150mg BID SR
Max:450mg/d IR and 400mg SR
Max one time dose=150mg IR and 200mg SR
SR does NOT allow for once a day dosing</td><td>Half-life: 12 hours

Active and Inactive metabolites</td><td>Over stimulation, headache, insomnia, nausea, agitation
High doses may cause psychotic symptoms
Little to no sexual dysfunction
Photosensitivity
Not for panic disorder</td></tr>
</table>

Adapted from references [2 - 4]

*Anticholinergic Side Effects: blurred vision, constipation, decreased salivation, delirium, hyperthermia, decreased sweating, memory problems, sinus tachycardia, delayed or retrograde ejaculation, erectile dysfunction, photophobia, urinary retention, decreased bronchial secretions, exacerbation of glaucoma

**Antihistaminergic Side Effects: sedation, weight gain, hypotension, nausea, vomiting, diarrhea, GI distress, constipation, dizziness

***Antiadrenergic Side Effects: postural hypotension (α_1), dizziness (α_1), headache, drowsiness, nausea, ejaculatory problems (α_1), erectile dysfunction, priapism, reflex tachycardia (α_1)

Atypical/Typical Antipsychotics

Target: psychotic symptoms, mood swings, acute mania, impulsivity, aggression

- Caution in hallucinogen-induced flash-backs, may make them worse.
- Side Effects vary, metabolic syndrome *versus* the risk of extrapyramidal side effects and tardive dyskinesia. The risks and benefits need to be clearly explained to the patient so they can make an educated decision.
- All carry a black box warning regarding an increased risk of death/cardio-vascular adverse reactions (stroke) in dementia related psychosis/use with caution in the elderly.

Dosing

Overall: Start low and titrate as needed, target the lowest effective dose. Use them for the shortest time necessary for substance induced symptoms.

Choice is largely empirical except for patient / medication considerations.

Table 4. Selected antipsychotic agents.

Medication	Daily Dosing Range	Pharmacokinetics	Side Effects
Haloperidol (Haldol)	0.5-20mg Oral tablet, solution, IM IM dose is ½ the oral dose	Half-life: 24 hours	High EPSE Low anticholinergic, antihistaminergic, and antiadrenergic NMS and TD Boxed warning for elderly
Loxapine (Loxitane)	10mg – 200mg Oral	Half-life: 24 hours	Less EPSE than haloperidol Moderate antiadrenergic, antihistaminergic, anticholinergic NMS and TD Boxed warning for elderly
Risperidone (Risperdal)	0.5 – 6mg Oral tablet, solution, M-Tab	Half-life: 24 hours CYP 2D6 primary metabolic route less *via* 3A4	Common: Antiadrenergic, antihistaminergic, Little to No anticholinergic activity Less Common: EPSE (dose related: increased risk as increase the dose), moderate hyperprolactinemia but less than traditional agents, weight gain, hyperlipidemia, hyperglycemia, stroke Rare: NMS, TD Boxed warning for elderly

(Table 4) contd.....

Medication	Daily Dosing Range	Pharmacokinetics	Side Effects
Quetiapine (Seroquel)	50-800mg divided BID start low and titrate up Elderly low 12.5-25mg HS or divided Lower doses – Antianxiety Medium – Bipolar Higher doses – Psychosis	Half-life: 12 hours but can be dosed all at bedtime CYP 3A4 primary metabolic route	Common: Antiadrenergic, antihistaminergic, little to no anticholinergic activity Less Common: mild elevation of ALT and AST, weight gain, hyperlipidemia, hyperglycemia, stroke Rare: EPSE, TD, NMS, glaucoma, mild hyperprolactinemia, prolonged QTc Boxed warning for elderly
Olanzapine (Zyprexa)	5-20mg	Half-life = 24 hours Metabolic route: CYP 1A2 – level decreased by smoking	Common: Antihistaminergic, anticholinergic, antiadrenergic, weight gain, hyperlipidemia, hyperglycemia Less Common: agitation, mild hyperprolactinemia, EPSE (dose related, less than risperidone), stroke Rare: NMS, TD Boxed warning for elderly
Aripiprazole (Abilify)	2-30 mg/day	Half-life = 72 hours CYP 3A4, 2D6 primary metabolic route	Common: Orthostatic hypotension, tremor, headache, insomnia, sedation Less Common: weight gain/loss, hyperlipidemia, hyperglycemia, stroke Rare: NMS, TD, hyperprolactinemia Boxed warning for elderly
Lurasidone (Latuda)	40 – 80mg once daily with food	Half-life: 18 hours Metabolic route: CYP 3A4 Moderately blocks alpha2C- and alpha2A Partial agonist at 5-HT1A Low to no blockade of H1 and M1	Common: restlessness, nausea, tremors, slow movement, muscle stiffness, and agitation Boxed warning for elderly

TD = Tardive Dyskinesia; NMS = Neuroleptic Malignant Syndrome; EPSE: Extra-pyramidal Side Effects. Adapted from references [2, 3]

Monitoring

Abnormal Involuntary Movement Scale (AIMS): baseline then every 6 months to a year.

Table 5. Metabolic monitoring.

	Baseline	12 Weeks	Quarterly	Annually
Personal/Family Hx	X			
Weight	X	X	X	
Blood Pressure	X	X		X
Fasting Plasma Glucose	X	X		X
Fasting Lipid Profile	X	X		X

Adapted from references [5, 6]

Additional Monitoring Recommended

Basal Metabolic Index - calculate when weighed

Waist measurement – baseline and 12 weeks then quarterly to every 6 months

HgbA1c if patient is already pre-diabetic or diabetic – with FPG

Other Side Effects

- Prolactin level elevation with high potency agents: traditional agents > risperidone > olanzapine > remaining atypicals > clozapine
- Seizures: occur in < 2% patients taking antipsychotics. Increased risk with sudden dose changes and abrupt DC. Unlikely to cause seizures in patients without a preexisting seizure disorder and patients on adequate anticonvulsant therapy.
  Relative risk: chlorpromazine > perphenazine, fluphenazine, trifluperazine, loxapine > thiothixene > haloperidol
- Relative Risk of QTc Prolongation with Antipsychotic Medications
  High: thioridazine (avoid), chlorpromazine, ziprasidone
  Mid: risperidone, quetiapine, clozapine, olanzapine, perphenazine
  Low: aripiprazole, lurasidone, paliperidone, oral haloperidol, oral fluphenazine
- Risk of Weight Gain (> 7%): Greatest to Least: clozapine >> olanzapine >> quetiapine = iloperidone = asenapine = risperidone > paliperidone = aripiprazole = ziprasidone = lurasidone

Extrapyramidal Side Effects (EPSE)

***Early Onset EPSE*:** Usually occur within the first four weeks of treatment.

Akathisia: Subjective feeling of motor restlessness, internal feeling of restlessness, feeling as if one has to move continuously.

Dystonic Reactions: Involuntary tonic contractions, may involve nearly any striatal muscle group. Most commonly involves head, face, and neck but may involve trunk, arms and legs. May occur abruptly or in an on and off again fashion over hours. Usually occur once but may reoccur with dosage increases.

Pseudo-Parkinsonism: Presentation of symptoms similar to those seen in Parkinson's Disease (bradykinesia, masked facies, shuffling gait, cog-wheel rigidity, akinesia, drooling, tremor, *etc.*).

***Late Onset EPSE*:** Typically occurs after six months or more of treatment, insidious.

Tardive Dyskinesia: Involuntary movements of the mouth, lips and tongue, may involve movements of the hands, feet, arms, legs and trunk. Choreiform movements are purposeless, involuntary and quick, while athetoid movements are continuous slow wave like movements usually in the distal portions of the extremities.

Course: EPSE may wax and wane over time, disappear during sleep, exacerbated by stress and emotional situations.

Treatment of Early - EPSE

Dystonias and Pseudoparkinsonism

Anticholinergic Medications: Drugs of Choice

Use when symptoms appear continue for 1 - 2 months then taper and re-evaluate need. Use smallest amount for shortest amount of time.

Prophylactic use only if it is known patient has developed EPSE in the past.

<u>Anticholinergic Agents</u>

- Start with lowest doses and titrate to effect.
  Benztropine Mesylate (Cogentin) 1 - 6mg PO or IM once daily or in divided doses.
  Diphenhydramine (Benadryl) 25 - 200mg PO or IM daily in divided doses.
- For Acute Dystonic Reactions - Use IM Anticholinergic.
  Usually see relief of dystonias in 1-2 minutes, repeat dose in 5 minutes if no relief occurs with first injection, it may take up to 40 minutes to resolve:
  Cogentin 1 - 2mg IM
  Benadryl 25 - 50mg IM

Akathisia

Propranolol (Inderal) 10mg BID initially, increase as needed and tolerated. Monitor vital signs. Caution in diabetes and asthma.

Benzodiazepines may also be effective for akathisia.

Treatment of Tardive Dyskinesia

Discontinue the current agent slowly over several weeks. Consider initiating Vitamin E 400-800IU. TD movements may initially worsen then improve. After 6 months off of the causative agent any residual movement may be permanent.

Clozapine (Clozaril) is the best antipsychotic at this time. Quetiapine is next.

Neuroleptic Malignancy Syndrome (NMS)

NMS is a potentially life threatening idiosyncratic reaction that develops over a 72 hour time period. Have a patient report any new onset high fever (> 104F) and the symptoms below. NMS can be seen with ALL antipsychotic medications.

Symptom Quad: Altered Mental Status, Lead Pipe Rigidity, Hyperthermia, Autonomic Instability

* May not see all 4 symptoms, look for gradients and combinations, atypical agents especially clozapine may not demonstrate this degree of stiffness as a

symptom.

Laboratories: VS, Temperature, highly elevated CPK (in the thousands), CBC with Diff (elevated WBC).

NMS Treatment: Aggressiveness depends upon patient clinical picture.

1. Discontinue antipsychotic medication.
2. Discontinue any anticholinergic medications.
3. Push fluids oral or intravenous depending on patient status.
4. Cool the patient down: Antipyretics, cooling blankets....
5. Symptomatic treatment: muscle relaxants, anxiolytics, dopaminergic agents.

If symptoms are severe go to Emergency Room or call 911.

Mood Stabilizers

Anticonvulsants

Targets: mood swings, withdrawal, anxiety, anger, impulsivity, aggression

- In certain situations some anticonvulsants may be useful in the detoxification and management of withdrawal syndromes.
- Antipsychotics may be of use in acute situations. Atypical agents have mood stabilizing abilities.

Table 6. Selected mood stabilizers.

Agent	Dosing	Pharmacokinetics and Pharmacology	Side Effects / Drug Interactions
Valproic Acid (Depakote, Depakene)	Initial dosing: 250mg BID or 500mg HS Can bolus 20-30 mg/kg in divided doses Dosed to effect and blood level MAX: 60mg/kg/day	Half-life = 12 hours No active metabolites Blood Level: 50-140 mg/L Minimal Lab Before: Baseline liver function test PG Test – Category X Birth Control recommended	Common: sedation, nausea, indigestion, diarrhea, tremor, weight gain Less Common: alopecia, rash, elevated LFTs (3x normal = monitor, 5x normal = DC) Rare: Suicidal thoughts Severe: hepatotoxicity, thrombocytopenia Interactions with other anticonvulsants

(Table 6) contd.....

Agent	Dosing	Pharmacokinetics and Pharmacology	Side Effects / Drug Interactions
Lamotrigine (Lamictal)	Dosing: 25mg HS for two weeks, increase to 50mg HS for two weeks, then increase to 100mg week 5, to 200mg in week 6 (target dose) Slower dosing if also on VPA Max: 500mg	Half-life = 24 hours	Sedation, headache, nausea, dizziness, diplopia, ataxia, blurred vision Rash (large %), decreased risk if increase dose slowly, dc drug if rash occurs Rare: Suicidal thoughts Ethinyl estradiol (OCs) decreases lamotrigine levels
Topiramate (Topamax)	Initial: 50mg/d Increase slowly (50mg/week) to target 200-400mg (div. BID)	Half-life = 24 hours Little hepatic metabolism primarily renal elimination	Sedation, ataxia, cognitive disturbance, paresthesias, weight loss, diarrhea, *kidney stones* Rare: Suicidal thoughts Inhibits some of the carbonic anhydrase enzymes (CA-II, CA-IV) Decreased digoxin, and estrogen (OC) levels Monitor: baseline and periodic bicarbonate levels
Carbamazepine (Tegretol)	Initial dosing: 200mg BID Maintenance: 600 - 800 mg BID	Half-life = 12 hours Blood Level: 6 -12 mg/L - AM trough Induces CYP 3A4 Autoinduction – starts in the first two weeks stable by week 4 Active metabolite Baseline LFTs, CBC with diff and periodic	Common: sedation, blurred vision, dizziness, insomnia, nausea, headache, rash, dry mouth, diplopia, Less Common: confusion, fatigue, impotence, rash, hyponatremia, urticaria, photosensitivity reaction, abnormal LFTs, Severe: Aplastic anemia, arrhythmias Rare: Suicidal thoughts
Gabapentin (Neurontin)	Initial dose:100mg TID titrate to effect on anxiety, QHS for sleep Max: 3600mg/day	Half-life = 6-8 hours Renal elimination	Common: sedation, Rare: suicidal thoughts * Not a great mood stabilizer, used off label for anxiety and sleep

Adapted from references [2, 3]

Management of Insomnia

The inability to sleep can be one of the primary reasons for relapse to the use of substances. It is important to treat it aggressively and with medications that do not promote relapse. Sleep hygiene should be strongly encouraged (Box 1). Cognitive behavioral therapy for insomnia can be highly effective.

Box 1: Sleep Hygiene

1. Get up at the same time every day – rising at a consistent time is the most important factor. Going to bed at the same time is also important.
2. Control your bedroom sleeping environment

    Adjust the temperature: cold, hot, fans, blankets, *etc.*
    Set the lighting: absolute dark, twilight, light
    Sound: absolute quiet (ear plugs), radio – calming music, white noise machine
    Get rid of distractions: NO computer, TV, desk (things you need to do), reading
    Turn your clock to face away from the bed (the alarm will still go off)

3. Develop a Bedtime Ritual

    Keep lights dim
    Make a to do list for the next day to clear the mind - after evening meal before bedtime
    Read something boring or calming
    Relaxation therapies: Meditation, progressive muscle relaxation, positive imagery
    Sip a cup of sedating/calming teas or warm milk

4. Limit activity in the bedroom to sleep and sex
5. No alcohol, caffeine or nicotine
6. Exercise in the morning, mid-day or right after supper. Not before bedtime.
7. Eat evening meal no later than 8:00PM. If tolerated, a small snack of high tryptophan foods at bedtime (warm milk, eggs, tuna fish, cottage cheese, soy beans, cashews, chicken and turkey - especially dark meat) may assist with sleep.

(Box 1) contd.....

8. NO naps. Some people can take a 20 minute power nap and wake refreshed. If a short nap invigorates you okay. If not, NO naps. No naps even powernaps after 3pm.
9. Sleep only when sleepy. Sleep as much as you need but no more.
10. If you can't sleep within 10-15 minutes, get up get out of bed and do something boring, music, read, no TV or computer, keep environment dimly lit. Once you feel sleepy go right back to bed.
11. If you wake up early in the morning with less than two hours before your alarm – stay up. Go to bed at the regular time.

Table 7. Selected agents for sleep.

Agent FDA Approved	Therapeutic Use	Dosing	Side Effects / Comments
Non-benzodiazepine Hypnotics Zolpidem (Ambien) Zaleplon (Sonata) Eszopiclone (Lunesta)	Insomnia Difficulty falling asleep (DFA) and Midnight awakening (MNA) DFA Insomnia	 Ambien: 2.5-5mg women 5-10mg men Max rec dose: 20mg Half-life = 3-4 hours Sonata: 5-10mg Max rec dose: 20mg Half-life = 1 hour May re-dose both agents if awake before 0100. Incr. chance am hangover 2-3mg	Common: headache, nausea, dizziness Large Doses (> 40mg/d): memory impairment, hangover, amnesia, ataxia OD: Tx flumazenil Other: No rebound insomnia or amnesia at therapeutic doses W/D: minor fatigue, nausea, slushing, stomach cramps will chronic high dose abrupt DC (higher than recommended doses. Possible incr. risk with Ambien) FDA warning regarding daytime impairment with zolpidem, most likely applies to all agents

(Table 7) contd.....

Agent FDA Approved	Therapeutic Use	Dosing	Side Effects / Comments
Ramelteon (Rozerem)	Sleep	8 mg 30 minutes before bedtime May need to go to 16mg (off label) Half-life = 1-2.6 hours Do not take with or immediately after a high fat meal	Common: somnolence, dizziness, nausea, headache Melatonin MT1 and MT2 receptor agonist
Doxepin	Sedative	3-6mg 30 minutes before bedtime	Low doses is antihistaminergic selective, higher doses add anticholinergic and antiadrenergic effects
<u>Antihistamines</u> Diphenhydramine (Benadryl) Hydroxyzine (Vistaril, Atarax) Cyproheptadine (Periactin)	Sedative Hypnotic	100-200mg/d 50-100mg/d 8-16 mg/d PTSD nightmares	Anticholinergic and antihistaminergic side effects Tolerance develops Cyproheptadine has anti-serotonergic properties – may interfere with effect of serotonergic agents
Off Label Use and Over-the-Counter			
Prazosin (Minipress)	PTSD associated dreams/ Nightmares	1-12mg daily, HS or divided doses, 20mg max Half-life = 2-4 hours	Common: Hypotension, Lightheadedness, Palpitations Constipation, Diarrhea, Nausea, Vomiting, Dizziness, Headache, Somnolence, Increased frequency of urination
Trazodone (Desyrel)	Depression, Insomnia *Watch for serotonin syndromes at doses > 200mg/day when used with SSRIs	Initial dose: 25 mg a day Primary use: SLEEP Maintenance for sleep: 50 - 150mg HS Depression: 200mg BID Max: 600mg	High alpha-adrenergic blockade results in high incidence of orthostatic hypotension Very Sedating Priapism - rare, urologic emergency

(Table 7) contd.....

Agent FDA Approved	Therapeutic Use	Dosing	Side Effects / Comments
Melatonin	Insomnia	Few adverse effects at doses < 10mg Minor side effects with these doses include: heavy head, headache	Insomnia: 0.3 to 10 mg administered one hour before sleep. Try different dosing times *i.e.* after the evening meal and titrating doses
Chamomile *(Matricaria recutita Chamaemelum nobile)*	Internal: GI spasm and inflammatory diseases, Menstrual cramps, anti-anxiety, sedation, Colic External: Eczema, Wound healing	GI problems and Anxiety: Tea three to four times a day – 1-2 teabags/cup of hot water Take on an empty stomach / between meals. Sleep: use a stronger tea (3-4 bags/cup) Children less than 2 years of age for colic use weak tea, small amounts	Rare cross reactivity with ragweed allergy. (swish and spit test: make a strong cup of tea, swish cool tea in mouth and spit. If your mouth is tingly and itchy do NOT use chamomile. Caution: NOT for use in large doses during pregnancy. Normal doses *not* considered a danger. Potential additive blood thinning.
Valerian (*Valeriana officinalis*)	Sedative-hypnotic, Antispasmodic	Standardized form: 0.5% essential oil Dosing: 500-1000mg at bedtime in capsule or tablet form. Additional doses (200-300mg) can be added during the day for anxiety	Mild with no am hangover Excessive initial doses (person dependent) may cause excitation, Monitor LFTs if used in large doses for long periods of time Caution: Data in pregnancy scarce, do not recommend use at this time.

* Lower potential for abuse *versus* benzodiazepines but it can be an issue. (Adapted from references [2, 3, 8 - 11]).

SUMMARY

Optimal management of co-morbid psychiatric and medical diagnoses while treating a substance use disorder is encouraged for best outcomes. Untreated symptoms may drive substance use in an effort to self-medicate.

Matching the patient and medication parameters can provide information for optimal medication selection. Patient finances and insurance issues also need to be taken into consideration. For each class of medications there is no superior product with the exception of clozapine in the antipsychotic category.

Optimize the dose with the target of symptom remission. Give enough medication for a long enough amount of time. Monitor symptoms and side effects frequently. Monitor for new onset thoughts of suicide at all visits, especially when using antidepressants and anticonvulsants.

PATIENT INFORMATION – MEDICATIONS FOR SUBSTANCE USE DISORDERS

What Medications can be Used to Treat Substance Use Disorders?

There are no medications that treat substance use disorders. However there are medications that can be used to help with withdrawal symptoms, cravings and other problems people face when dealing with their substance. We also use medications to treat any underlying medical or psychiatric problem.

There are medications that can be prescribed as substitute therapy for opioid use disorder. And specific medications are used in alcohol use disorder to help with managing craving and the impulsive use of alcohol.

Are these Medications Addictive?

The majority of medications used for these disorders are not addictive. Occasionally medications that have the potential for misuse are prescribed for short-term problems and in some individual instances longer. In these instances medication use must be closely monitored and re-evaluated.

Are there Side Effects Associated with these Medications?

All medications are associated with side effects. If your provider determines a medication is right for you, discuss the specific side effects of the recommended medication with them. Ask if there are alternatives to that medication if those side effects concern you.

Specific patient information on medications can be found at NAMI.org, the website for the National Alliance on Mental Illness. You can find information on the internet as well.

Do I Need to Take these Medications for a Long Time?

If the medication is prescribed for an underlying medical or psychiatric diagnosis, that issue may require long term treatment. You will need to discuss this with your provider to determine the best course of action for you.

What Non-drug therapies are Available for Substance Use Disorders?

Group therapies such as Alcoholics Anonymous (AA), Narcotics Anonymous (NA) and others provide support for maintaining sobriety, inpatient and outpatient substance treatment programs, and one-on-one meetings with a provider or therapist can be of assistance in managing substance use disorders and psychiatric illnesses. Generally people use a combination of these options.

CONFLICT OF INTEREST

The author confirms that she has no conflict of interest to declare for this publication.

ACKNOWLEDGEMENTS

Declared none.

REFERENCES

[1] Lingford-Hughes AR, Welch S, Peters L, Nutt DJ. BAP updated guidelines: evidence-based guidelines for the pharmacological management of substance abuse, harmful use, addiction and comorbidity: recommendations from BAP. J Psychopharmacol (Oxford) 2012; 26(7): 899-952. [http://dx.doi.org/10.1177/0269881112444324] [PMID: 22628390]

[2] Stahl SM. Essential psychopharmacology: the prescriber's guide. 2nd ed., New York: Cambridge University Press 2006.

[3] Stahl SM. stahl's essential psychopharmacology: neuroscientific basis and practical applications. 3rd ed., New York: Cambridge University Press 2008.

[4] Qaseem A, Snow V, Denberg TD, Forciea MA, Owens DK. Using second-generation antidepressants to treat depressive disorders: a clinical practice guideline from the American College of Physicians. Ann Intern Med 2008; 149(10): 725-33. [http://dx.doi.org/10.7326/0003-4819-149-10-200811180-00007] [PMID: 19017591]

[5] Hasnain M, Vieweg WV, Fredrickson SK, Beatty-Brooks M, Fernandez A, Pandurangi AK. Clinical

monitoring and management of the metabolic syndrome in patients receiving atypical antipsychotic medications. Prim Care Diabetes 2009; 3(1): 5-15.
[http://dx.doi.org/10.1016/j.pcd.2008.10.005] [PMID: 19083283]

[6] American Psychiatric Association, American Association of Clinical Endocrinologists, North American Association for the Study of Obesity. Consensus devel-opment conference on antipsychotic drugs and obesity and diabetes. Diabetes Care 2004; 27(2): 596-601.
[PMID: 14747245]

[7] Wenzel-Seifert K, Wittmann M, Haen E. QTc prolongation by psychotropic drugs and the risk of Torsade de Pointes. Dtsch Arztebl Int 2011; 108(41): 687-93. [cited: 5th June 2013].
[PMID: 22114630]

[8] Ringdahl EN, Pereira SL, Delzell JE Jr. Treatment of primary insomnia. J Am Board Fam Pract 2004; 17(3): 212-9. [cited: 1st Aug 2013].
[http://dx.doi.org/10.3122/jabfm.17.3.212] [PMID: 15226287]

[9] Roth T, Stubbs C, Walsh JK. Ramelteon (TAK-375), a selective MT1/MT2-receptor agonist, reduces latency to persistent sleep in a model of transient insomnia related to a novel sleep environment. Sleep 2005; 28(3): 303-7.
[PMID: 16173650]

[10] Simpson TL, Saxon AJ, Meredith CW, *et al.* A pilot trial of the alpha-1 adrenergic antagonist, prazosin, for alcohol dependence. Alcohol Clin Exp Res 2009; 33(2): 255-63.
[http://dx.doi.org/10.1111/j.1530-0277.2008.00807.x] [PMID: 18945226]

[11] Brower KJ, Conroy DA, Kurth ME, Anderson BJ, Stein MD. Ramelteon and improved insomnia in alcohol-dependent patients: a case series. J Clin Sleep Med 2011; 7(3): 274-5.
[PMID: 21677897]

CHAPTER 6

Motivational Interviewing

Imad Alsakaf[1,*], Subhash C. Bhatia[2] and Shashi K. Bhatia[3]

[1] *Creighton University School of Medicine 3528 Dodge Street Omaha, NE 68131 USA*

[2] *Department of Psychiatry, Mental Health and Behavioral Sciences, Creighton University; Department VA Nebraska- Western Iowa Health Care System 4101 Woolworth Ave Omaha, NE 68105, USA*

[3] *Departments of Psychiatry and Pediatrics, Division of Child and Adolescent Psychiatry, Creighton University, 3528 Dodge Omaha, NE 68131, USA*

Abstract: Motivational interviewing (MI) is to motivate patients with addictive and non-addictive disorders like noncompliant patients, to help them develop skills to find intrinsic motivation for change through resolution of ambivalence . Ambivalence may lead to arguments against change referred to as sustain talk. Strategies to decrease sustain talk may promote change talk. These strategies include: straight reflection, amplified reflection, double sided reflection, emphasizing autonomy, agreeing with a twist, reframing, running head start, and coming along side. Five principles for creating condition for change are: expressing empathy, avoiding confrontation, supporting self-efficacy, rolling with resistance, and developing discrepancy between the patient's behavior and his/her own goals and values. Key skills needed for MI include: open ended questioning, reflective listening, affirmations, periodic summarization of the content of the session, and informing and advising with permission of patient. The successful therapeutic process for MI involves: establishing rapport, setting the agenda, assessing readiness for change, sharpening the focus to what the patient truly wants to change, identifying ambivalence, eliciting self-motivating statements, handling resistance, and shifting focus of conversation to get around resistance. The stages of change model is distinct from MI but naturally fit together. MI helps patients move from one stage of change to another *e.g.* from pre-contemplation, contemplation, preparation, action, to maintenance.

[*] **Corresponding author Imad Alsakaf:** Creighton University School of Medicine 3528 Dodge Street Omaha, NE 68131 USA; Tel: 402-572-2483; Fax: 402-572-3472; E-mail: imadalsakaf@creighton.edu

Subhash C. Bhatia (Ed.)

Keywords: Affirmation, Ambivalence, Change talk, Commitment, Developing discrepancy, Empathy, Motivational interviewing, Open-ended questions, Reflective listening, Rolling with resistance, Self-motivating statements, Stages of change, Summarization, Sustain talk.

KEY LEARNING POINTS

1. Motivational Interviewing uses non-judgmental, non-confrontational, and a non-adversarial approach to help patient mobilize motivation to change behavior.
2. This change is through a focused and goal directed counseling by exploration and resolution of ambivalence.
3. This counseling involves open ended questioning, reflective listening, affirmations and periodic summarization of sessions.
4. The patient is made aware of behaviors and their consequences, is engaged in change talk and helped to mobilize intrinsic, not imposed, motivation for such a change.

BACKGROUND

Miller and Rollnick provide a technical definition of Motivational Interviewing (MI) where MI is considered a specific type of communication that is goal oriented and collaborative in nature with emphasis on language that leads to change. MI is intended to support personal drive for and commitment to change in a particular way by provoking and examining the individual's specific motivation for change, and it is conducted in a way that conveys empathy and nonjudgmental acceptance [1]. Even though this technique was specifically developed for patients with addictive disorders, it can be adapted for situations outside the field of addiction, for example, to increase patients' motivation for adherence to medical or mental health treatments, health promotion, problem gambling and dual diagnosis *etc*. This is supported by over 200 randomized clinical trials [2]. Highly interactive MI groups can also mobilize motivation to change [3].

PROCESS

MI theorists hold that MI is about aiding people resolve their ambivalence (indecision or fluctuation where one feels two ways about an idea, feeling or action) in a specific trend of change. When a therapist pushes for change with an ambivalent individual, it results in the other person providing opposite arguments. Arguments against change are referred to as *sustain talk*. That is why, in MI, the interviewer tries to elicit *change talk* (self-motivating speech) from within the individual, and to strengthen that change talk. People are more likely to get convinced by what they themselves say. MI is not about forcing or tricking people to change. In other words, MI is a facilitative style to communication that induces natural change [1].

As part of MI, sustain talk is a normal aspect of ambivalence and should not be considered as resistance [1]. One can respond to sustain talk in ways that could increase or decrease it. There are various ways to respond to sustain talk that could result in its decrease and may promote change talk [1]. The strategies to accomplish this may include: (a) *straight reflection*, simple or complex reflective statements can sometimes promote change talk (b) *amplified reflection,* the reflective statement with the intention to exaggerate what the individual has said (c) *double sided reflection*, reflective statement recognizes both the sustain talk and change talk that was previously expressed by the individual (d) *emphasizing autonomy* which makes it easier for people to choose change, (e) *reframing* or providing a different perspective for what the patient is sharing (f) *agreeing with a twist*, a combination of both reflection and reframing (g) *running head start*: The purpose here is to hear out the main drives for motivations for unwillingness when change talk is not provided, and then to ask about the negative attributes of the current situation and the benefits of changing the target behavior (h) *coming along side*: this is used when all attempts fail to elicit change talk. Joining with the individual's sustain talk will occasionally induce some change talk.

There are five principles for creating condition for change. These are:

1. Express empathy by sharing an informed understanding of a person's ambivalence and reasons for hesitation.
2. Avoid arguments or confrontation and allow patient to hear themselves. This will decrease resistance to change.
3. Support self-efficacy by encouraging the patient to make positive statements

which demonstrate self-efficacy. Negative statements can be reframed for example rather than saying "I am a loser" it can be reframed such that the patient may say "I know what I need to do to succeed".

4. Roll with the resistance may involve asking for clarification of a statement and having the patient see the discrepancy from where they are and where they should be.
5. Developing discrepancy involves establishing realistic goals, making the patient realize the difference between current and ideal goals where one is now and where he/she should be, generates discrepancy and creates conditions for change. Discrepancy between a core value and a specific behavior can be a significant motivator for change when explored in a supportive manner [1].

The successful therapeutic process for MI involves 8 steps [4]:

1. Establishing rapport by consistently being genuine to develop trust.
2. Patient setting the agenda based on his or her priorities.
3. Assessing readiness for change by asking a patient on a 1-10 point scale "Where are you for making a change?"
4. Sharpening the focus to what the patient truly wants to change.
5. Identifying ambivalence by asking patient points for and against change.
6. Eliciting self-motivating statements by asking what will be the best outcome for changing this situation and have them rephrase communication in a positive way.
7. Handling resistance by reflecting and sharing in a clear way what you are hearing, avoiding confrontation and using humor.
8. Shifting the focus of conversation to get around resistance.

The four key aspects that underlie MI are *partnership*, *acceptance*, *compassion* and *evocation* [1].

Since people are the undisputed experts on themselves, MI considers *partnership* as an important aspect of the spirit of MI. The therapeutic relationship is an active collaboration between two experts: the patient and the therapist [1]. *Acceptance* includes the following four aspects: absolute worth, accurate empathy, autonomy support, and affirmation. Acceptance involves valuing the inherent worth and potential of the patient, showing an active interest in trying to understand the patient's internal perspectives, honoring and respecting the patient's irrevocable right as well as capacity of self-directions, and seeking and acknowledging his/her strengths [1].

Compassion represents an intentional commitment to pursue the best interests of the patient [1]. In MI premise is that people already have within them what they need and have qualities to achieve positive changes. The task of the therapist is to evoke these positive qualities or to call them forth [1].

There are four overlapping processes in MI: *Engaging*, *focusing*, *evoking*, and *planning*. Engaging is the process by which the therapist and the patient establish a beneficial connection and a working relationship. In the process of engaging the therapist and the patient increases focus on a specific agenda. With change in one or more particular area as a focus, the next process in MI is *evoking*, which involves eliciting the client's motivation to achieve the specific change(s). When people are motivated enough to reach the threshold of readiness to change, they begin thinking about when and how to change rather than whether or why to change [1].

Core skills for MI

1. Ask open questions: The therapist needs to listen and to facilitate expression by having the patient to do most of the talking. One important skill to encourage the client to express himself/herself and to examine his/her concerns is to ask open-ended questions.
2. Listen reflectively: People don't always verbalize what they actually mean. The reflective listener formulate a guess as to what the intended meaning was, and then expressed this guess in the form of a statement. A statement is utilized, rather than a question, because a statement is less likely to induce resistance. Reflective listening is a method of checking, rather than presuming that you already aware of what is meant [1].
3. Affirm: Praise and expressing appreciation and understanding help the provider to establish a therapeutic relationship and to enhance the individual's self-exploration.

4. Summarize: Summary statements need to be used during MI to link and reinforce discussed subjects.
5. Inform and advise with permission of patient: It is important that the therapist does not provide unsolicited expert opinion. In MI, the therapist offers information or advice only when the patient is willing to receive that. It is important the therapist recognizes the patient's right to implement or not the therapist's advice, and to help the patient reach their own conclusions about the relevance of any information or advice to their own goal, perspectives and needs.

MOTIVATION ENHANCEMENT

There are 8 strategies to enhance motivation [5]. These include:

1. Giving advice about behaviors to be changed.
2. Removing barrier for access to help.
3. Providing choice "you have a right not to change or make change I am here to encourage change".
4. Decreasing the desirability of ambivalence in promoting change.
5. Practicing empathy by genuine understanding and reflection of the patient's predicament.
6. Providing feedback from collateral sources for the patient to get a full understanding of the situation.
7. Clarifying goals. Identifying the ideal goal and path to reach that goal.
8. Active help through coordination of care and showing real interest in having them obtain such care.

THE STAGES OF CHANGE

The stages of change model are distinct from MI, although they naturally fit together [6]. MI helps patients move from one stage of change to another. Prochaska and DiClemente described the following stages of change [7]:

1. Precontemplation: The patient is unaware of the problem or does not want to change it.
2. Contemplation: The patient is considering possibly making some changes.

3. Preparation: The patient is ready to make some change and develops a plan for that change.
4. Action: The patient acts upon his plan to change.
5. Maintenance: The patient works on sustaining the achieved change.

SUMMARY

MI skills involve: expression of empathy and reflective listening, noting discrepancy between current and desired behavior, avoiding argument and rolling with resistance, have the person believe in their ability to change, communicate respect and acceptance, establish non-judgmental collaborative relationship, be supportive and understanding, complimenting rather than criticizing, listening rather than telling, gently persuading the person to change, giving the person autonomy to change and providing support throughout the process of change and recovery [8].

MOTIVATIONAL INTERVIEW-PATIENT EDUCATION SHEET

What is Motivational Interview?

This is a talk therapy and technique of counseling which helps patients identify and change behaviors to promote recovery and healthy behaviors.

What are the Principles of this Therapy?

Empathy, non-argumentativeness, believing in a person's self-efficacy and ability to make change, not confronting resistance but rolling with it and developing awareness of consequences of the current situation and developing realistic goals and priorities for change.

How does MI Work?

The technique helps to make a person realize need or motivation to change, from within and through their own effort with support of the therapist. This is with an understanding that there is a cost for not changing and benefit to change. Based on this realization a person makes the change towards positive behaviors.

CONFLICT OF INTEREST

The authors confirm that they have no conflict of interest to declare for this publication.

ACKNOWLEDGEMENTS

Declared none.

REFERENCES

[1] Miller WR, Rollnick S. Motivational interviewing: helping people change. Third Edition., the Guilford Press 2013.

[2] Miller WR, Zweben A, DiClemente CC, Rychatarick RG. Motivational enhancement therapy manual. Washington, DC: National Institute on Alcohol Abuse and Alcoholism 1994.

[3] Wagner CC, Ingersoll KS, *et al.* Motivational interviewing in groups. New York: Guilford Press 2013. [http://dx.doi.org/10.1093/acrefore/9780199975839.013.252]

[4] Burke BL, Arkowitz H, Menchola M. The efficacy of motivational interviewing: a meta-analysis of controlled clinical trials. J Consult Clin Psychol 2003; 71(5): 843-61. [http://dx.doi.org/10.1037/0022-006X.71.5.843] [PMID: 14516234]

[5] Bundy C. Changing behaviour: using motivational interviewing techniques. J R Soc Med 2004; 97 (Suppl. 44): 43-7. [PMID: 15239293]

[6] Levounis P, Arnaout B. Handbook of motivation and change: a practical guide for clinicians. American Psychiatric Publishing, Inc 2010.

[7] Prochaska JO, DiClemente CC. The transtheoretical approach: crossing traditional boundaries of therapy. Homewood, IL: Dow Jones-Irwin 1984.

[8] http://www.sampsa.gov/co-occuring/topics/training/skills.aspx , [accessed November 11, 2013];

CHAPTER 7

Alcohol Use Disorders

Teri Gabel[1,*] and **Sidney Kauzlarich**[2]

[1] *VA Nebraska Western Iowa Health Care System, Clinical Pharmacy Specialist - Mental Health, Omaha, NE 68105; Department of Psychiatry, University Of Nebraska College of Medicine Omaha NE 68198; Drug Therapy Consultants, PC 5116 N 116 St, Omaha NE 68164 USA*

[2] *Douglas County Community Mental Health Center, 4102 Woolworth Ave, Omaha, NE 68105 USA*

Abstract: This chapter reviews the epidemiology and pathophysiology of alcohol use disorders. No two patients with alcohol use disorders are the same and recognition of these patients in our practice is the first priority. Diagnostic indicators and the CAGE questions that can be used to assist in the identification of patients with alcohol use disorders are presented. Non-drug therapies are integral and include lifestyle changes, group therapies (alcoholics anonymous), and individual therapies (*i.e.*, cognitive behavioral therapy). These and other non-drug treatment options are discussed in this chapter. Medication options for the management of outpatient alcohol withdrawal are discussed and include benzodiazepines and anticonvulsant agents (off-label use). Medications to assist in maintaining sobriety and reduce craving should be offered to all patients. Medications discussed in this chapter include acamprosate, naltrexone and disulfiram. The information presented includes discussion of patient specific characteristics such as renal and hepatic function and underlying psychiatric issues such as anxiety, depression and insomnia that may affect medication selection and outcome. This chapter includes key learning points and a patient vignette to assist the learner. A patient education sheet on alcohol use disorders and additional patient resources accompanies the chapter.

Keywords: Acamprosate, Alcohol withdrawal, CAGE, Craving, Disulfiram, Naltrexone.

[*] **Corresponding author Teri Gabel:** VA Nebraska Western Iowa Health Care System, Clinical Pharmacy Specialist - Mental Health, Omaha, NE 68105; Department of Psychiatry, University Of Nebraska College of Medicine Omaha NE 68198; Drug Therapy Consultants, PC 5116 N 116 St, Omaha NE 68164 USA ; Tel: (402) 493-5222; Email: pharmdherb@gmail.com

Subhash C. Bhatia (Ed.)

KEY POINTS

1. No two patients with alcohol dependence are the same.
2. Non-drug therapies are an integral part of treatment.
3. Medications to assist in sobriety and reduce craving should be offered to all patients.
4. Acamprosate may target relief drinking.
5. Naltrexone may target impulse drinking.
6. Disulfiram is most effective when used in a program that observes individuals taking the medication.
7. Desire to quit affects the success of medication and treatment.

CLINICAL VIGNETTE

Karen is a 32 year old female that presented to her primary care physician with complaints of "stomach pain" and problems with "nervousness and insomnia". Further questioning reveals Karen has recently separated from her husband and about 6 weeks ago was fired from her job because of being under the influence of alcohol while at work.

Karen reports she started using alcohol at age 17 and received two "minor in possession" citations and was required to attend mandatory chemical dependency treatment at age 18. Karen states her parents allowed her to use alcohol during her teen years and reported both parents struggled with alcoholism. By age 25 Karen received 2 driving under the influence charges, and had lost 3 jobs because of alcohol consumption, and the subsequent hangovers which led to excessive absenteeism. Karen reports her husband has been encouraging her to seek treatment and he finally separated from her because he reports she is an "angry drunk".

Karen began drinking beer daily, but over the past 2 years she has been drinking about a 1/5th of vodka every day.

Karen now believes her alcohol use is a problem because her husband has left her, citing her alcohol use as the reason. Karen reports she stopped drinking about one week ago and notes the tremors and anxiety have decreased, but she continues to have problems with insomnia, anxiety and cravings for alcohol.

Karen's physical exam revealed an enlarged liver and lab work revealed elevated liver enzymes and a mean corpuscular volume greater than 100fl in an otherwise healthy appearing female.

The physician educated Karen regarding the undesirable effects of excessive alcohol use on mood, sleep, and anxiety, and also acknowledged and supported Karen's recent sobriety. The physician reviewed with Karen the risks and benefits of the available pharmacological treatments for alcoholism. This discussion included the risks of using medications during pregnancy and breast feeding. Karen was started on acamprosate and encouraged to attend Alcoholic Anonymous meetings on a daily basis.

INTRODUCTION

Alcohol Use Disorders (AUDs) can be devastating conditions that negatively impact every aspect of a person's life. Frequently, AUDs impair psychological, social, interpersonal, educational and occupational functioning. AUDs may also contribute to violence, legal problems, employment difficulties and significant family conflict. Furthermore, those individuals afflicted with AUDs suffer from increased medical and psychiatric morbidity.

AUDs are responsible for a remarkable toll on the United States economy. The overall annual cost related to AUDs approached $185 billion in 1998 [1]. Alcohol use has been attributed to more than 60 different medical conditions, and nearly 40 percent of hospitalized patients receive treatment for complications of alcohol misuse, which accounts for 15 percent of healthcare cost [2]. Individuals with alcohol-related medical illnesses have more frequent hospitalizations and longer hospital stays compared to individuals without AUDs [3]. Untreated alcoholic individuals have at least a 100 percent higher general health care cost compared to nonalcoholic individuals [4]. In 1998 expenditures for health care services to treat AUDs and the medical consequences of alcohol consumption was estimated to be $26.3 billion [5].

In the year 2000, alcohol use directly and indirectly accounted for approximately 85,000 preventable deaths in the United States. Only tobacco use and poor diet and physical inactivity surpassed alcohol use in preventable causes of death [6]. Each year up to 37 percent of rapes and sexual assaults, 27 percent of aggravated assaults and 15 percent of robberies involve the use of alcohol [4]. In addition, it is estimated that nearly 40 percent of all traffic fatalities are alcohol related and alcoholics are nearly five times more likely to die in a motor vehicle accident [4].

Epidemiology

According to the National Institute of Mental Health Epidemiologic Catchment Area Study (ECA) the lifetime prevalence of AUDs is about 13.5%. The National Institute on Alcohol Abuse and Alcoholism (NIAAA) conducted the National Epidemiologic Survey on Alcohol and Related Conditions (NESARC) from 2001 to 2002. This survey consisted of nearly 43000 face-to-face interviews. This study revealed that approximately 18 million adults in the United States suffer from AUDs [7]. This is an increase from the number reported in a survey conducted by NIAAA from 1991 to 1992, at which time 13.8 million adults suffered from AUDs [7]. Furthermore, the NESARC Survey found that approximately 8 million individuals in the United States are alcohol dependent [7].

Alcohol use frequently starts at an early age. According to the 2008 Monitoring the Future Data, nearly 17 percent of eighth graders, 30 percent of 10th graders and over 40 percent of 12th graders have used alcohol in the past 30 days [8]. The same survey indicates nearly 20 percent of 10th graders and about 30 percent of 12th graders had become intoxicated with alcohol within the past 30 days individuals that begin using alcohol before the age of 15 are four times more likely to develop alcoholism than those who begin using alcohol at age 21 [4].The prevalence of adult alcohol abuse declines as the age of first use rises. Nearly 14 percent of individuals who began drinking at age 14, are subsequently diagnosed with alcohol abuse, compared to only 2.5 percent of those who began drinking at age 25 and older [9]. Overall, the risk for lifetime alcohol abuse decreased by 8 percent with each increasing year of age of onset of drinking [9]. Alcohol use increases through the teen years, peaks in the early 20s, and tends to decline thereafter. Generally speaking, AUDs are most common between ages 18-29 and decline to its lowest prevalence in individuals aged 65 or older [7].

The NESARC Survey revealed that gender also influences the rate of AUDs. Males showed significantly higher rates of AUDs with alcohol abuse being nearly 7 percent for males compared to 2.55 percent for females. The rate of alcohol dependence for males was 5.42 percent and for females 2.32 percent. This gender difference holds true across cultures including Whites, Blacks, Asians, Native Americans and Hispanics [7].

The NESARC Survey also revealed ethnicity appears to play a significant role in determining AUDs. The prevalence of alcohol abuse was significantly greater among Whites (5.10 percent) compared to Hispanics (3.97 percent), Blacks (3.29 percent) and Asians (2.13 percent). The prevalence of alcohol dependence in Native Americans was highest at (6.35 percent), Hispanics (3.95 percent), Whites (3.83 percent), and Asians (2.41 percent) [6]. The NESARC Survey also uncovered a trend from 1991 to 2002 of increased rates of alcohol abuse by black males, Asian females and Hispanic males between ages of 18 to 29 [7].

The National Co-morbidity Survey (NCS) by Kessler *et al.* in 1996 and the Epidemiologic Catchment Area (ECA) study by Regier *et al.* in 1990 are two significant studies performed in the United States that evaluated the co-occurrence of AUDs and psychiatric disorders. The NCS revealed that 29.2 percent of study subjects with alcohol dependence had a co-occurring mood disorder. The NCS also indicated alcohol dependent individuals were 3.9 times more likely to have had a major depressive disorder (27.9 percent) during the previous year when compared to those who were not alcohol dependent. In addition, a diagnosis of bipolar disorder was shown to be 6.3 times more likely among alcohol dependent individuals compared to individuals without alcohol dependence.

NCS also revealed that 36.9 percent of individuals with alcohol dependence had a co-occurring anxiety disorder, including generalized anxiety disorder, post-traumatic stress disorder and panic disorder. According to the ECA Study, the lifetime prevalence of co-occurring schizophrenia in alcohol dependent individuals is estimated to be 24 percent. Therefore, alcohol dependent individuals are nearly four times more likely to suffer from schizophrenia than an individual without alcohol dependence. Please refer to Table **1** for more detailed results from the NCS and ECA Study.

Table 1. Prevalence of alcohol abuse and dependence.

Prevalence of Psychiatric Disorders in People with Alcohol Abuse and Alcohol Dependence				
Comorbid Disorder	**Alcohol abuse**		**Alcohol dependence**	
National Comorbidity Survey[1]	**1-year rate (%)**	**Odds ratio**	**1-year rate (%)**	**Odds ratio**
Mood disorders	12.3	1.1	29.2	3.6*
Major depressive disorder	11.3	1.1	27.9	3.9*
Bipolar disorder	0.3	0.7	1.9	6.3*
Anxiety disorders	29.1	1.7	36.9	2.6*
GAD	1.4	0.4	11.6	4.6*
Panic disorder	1.3	0.5	3.9	1.7
PTSD	5.6	1.5	7.7	2.2*
Epidemiologic Catchment Area[2] study	**Lifetime rate (%)**	**Odds ratio**	**Lifetime rate (%)**	**Odds ratio**
Schizophrenia	9.7	1.9	24	3.8

NOTES: * Odds ratio was significantly different from 1 at 0.05 levels. The odds ratio represents the increased chance that someone with alcohol abuse or dependence will have the comorbid psychiatric disorder (*e.g.*, a person with alcohol dependence is 3.6 times more likely to also have co-occurring mood disorder compared to a person without alcohol dependence).

The 1–year rate of a disorder reflects the percentage of people who met the criteria for the disorder during the year prior to the survey.

The lifetime rate reflects the percentage of people who met the criteria for the disorder at any time in their lifetime.

SOURCES: [1]Kessler *et al.* 1996. [2]Regier *et al.* 1990.

Furthermore, one needs to keep in mind the significant co-occurrence of antisocial personality disorder and AUDs. According to the NCS the lifetime prevalence of co-occurring alcohol dependence in individuals with antisocial personality disorders is nearly 16.9 percent for men, which is an odds ratio of greater than 8, and 7.8 percent for women with an odds ratio greater than 17. Lastly, individuals with alcohol dependence tend to have a high rate of co-occurring drug use disorders. NCS revealed that nearly 30 percent of alcohol dependent men and nearly 35 percent of alcohol dependent women had a co-occurring drug dependence problem.

Etiology

The etiology of AUDs involves a complex relationship between psychological, social, environmental and genetic factors. Although one cannot ignore the psychosocial and environmental influences, a great deal of research has been focused on the genetic causes for AUDs. Research indicates that AUDs are familial [10]. First degree relatives have a three to fourfold increase in prevalence of alcohol abuse compared to the general population [11]. Based on identical twin studies, genetic factors are estimated to account for 50 to 60 percent of the risk for developing alcohol abuse [10]. It has also been shown that children of alcohol dependent parents who are raised by non-alcohol dependent individuals remain at increased risk for an AUD [12, 13].

Diagnosis

The American Psychiatric Association's Diagnostic and Statistical Manual of Mental Disorders Fifth Edition (DSM-5) has classified Alcohol-Related Disorders into the following: Alcohol Use Disorder, Alcohol Intoxication, Alcohol Withdrawal, Other Alcohol-Induced Disorder and Unspecified Alcohol-Related Disorder.

According to the DSM-5 there is a cluster of 9 behaviors used to identify individuals with AUDs. These behaviors include consuming large amounts of alcohol or using alcohol for long periods of time; inability to decrease or stop alcohol use; spending significant periods of time obtaining, consuming and/or recovering from the effects of alcohol use; experiencing significant cravings for alcohol; use of alcohol is impairing social functioning; alcohol use is causing inability to complete responsibilities at home, work and/or school; alcohol use is interfering with recreational activities; using alcohol while engaged in potentially dangerous activities; alcohol use causing physical and emotional problems. In addition to these 9 behaviors physiological tolerance to alcohol and symptoms of alcohol withdrawal contribute to the diagnosis of AUDs.

The DSM 5 allows clinicians to specify how severe the substance use disorder is based on how many of the above criteria exist. Two or three criteria indicate a mild alcohol use disorder, four or five criteria indicate a moderate alcohol use disorder, and six or more criteria indicate a severe alcohol use disorder. Clinicians can also specify if the condition is "in early remission", "in sustained remission" and/or if the individual is "on medication maintenance therapy" and/or "in a controlled environment".

Alcohol is a widely used substance by individuals of all ages, gender and ethnicity and therefore the clinician should screen all individuals for an AUD. Individuals may worry about stigma and can be embarrassed by their drinking behavior and the consequences of their alcohol use. This fact, along with frequent use of the defense mechanism denial can make it very difficult to elicit accurate substance use histories from individuals suffering from AUDs. Frequently this can be overcome by using a nonjudgmental empathic approach to questioning along with interviewing family members and friends of the individual suspected of an AUD.

A simple and quick screening tool that can be used to help identify individuals that may require further evaluation for an AUD is the CAGE questionnaire. The questionnaire consists of the following four questions: Have you ever felt the need to cut down on drinking? Have you ever felt annoyed by criticism of your drinking? Have you ever had guilty feelings about your drinking? Do you ever take a morning eye opener (a drink first thing in the morning to steady your nerves or get rid of a hangover)? One yes response to any of the CAGE questions suggests the need for further assessment for an AUD. A yes response to 2 or 3 of the questions indicates a high index of suspicion for presence of an AUD. Responding with yes to all 4 questions is virtually diagnostic for alcohol dependence [14].

Obtaining a thorough substance use history, mental health history and medical history is imperative because physical examination and laboratory findings supporting a diagnosis of an AUD may be lacking early in the disease state. Given the familial nature of AUDs, a thorough family history of AUDs should also be explored. The clinician should inquire whether or not past or current use of alcohol has interfered with social, interpersonal, educational, psychological and/or occupational functioning. In addition, the clinician should inquire about accidents, injuries, medical and/or legal ramifications secondary to alcohol use.

Specifics about age of first alcohol use, frequency and quantity of current and past use should be investigated. The clinician also needs to search for evidence of physiological dependence on alcohol such as the need to increase the amount of alcohol consumed to achieve desired effects or the need to consume alcohol, or a similar substance, to prevent alcohol withdrawal symptoms.

When evaluating an individual one must remember alcohol can cause psychiatric conditions as well as exacerbate existing psychiatric disorders. According to the DSM-5 alcohol use can cause the following psychiatric conditions; alcohol induced mood, anxiety, sleep, and psychotic disorders. Alcohol has also been shown to cause significant cognitive disorders including dementia. Every individual presenting with a mental illness and/or cognitive impairment deserves a thorough evaluation for AUDs because of the high rate of co-occurance.

Individuals with AUDs can present with normal physical examination findings especially in the early stages of the disease. However, as the disease progresses and medical complications develop, physical examination findings and complaints of physical symptoms become more apparent and are usually secondary to the damaging effects of alcohol on organ systems. Alcohol can be toxic to nearly every organ system. However, the gastrointestinal system tends to be particularly vulnerable to the toxic effects of alcohol. It is common for patients with alcohol dependence to present with signs and symptoms of gastritis, peptic ulcer disease, acute and chronic pancreatitis, alcoholic hepatitis, cirrhosis, esophageal varices and gastrointestinal bleeding. Furthermore individuals with alcohol dependence are at increased risk for cancers of the oral cavity, pharynx, larynx, esophagus, colon, rectum, liver, pancreas, breast, and thyroid gland [15 - 17].

The central nervous system (CNS) is also vulnerable to the acute and chronic toxic effects of alcohol. Alcohol dependent individuals can present with a broad array of cognitive and neurological impairments including a history of black outs, memory and concentration problems, dementia, incoordination, problems with gait, and signs and symptoms of alcohol intoxication and withdrawal. Toxic effects of alcohol on the CNS can also result in sleep disturbances, depression, anxiety, and psychotic symptoms. Individuals with excessive alcohol use are also at increased risk for developing hypertension and alcoholic cardiomyopathy.

Laboratory tests can be helpful in identifying and monitoring individuals with alcohol dependence. However one should not rely too heavily on biomarkers to make a diagnosis of alcohol dependence because many alcohol dependent individuals present with normal lab findings. Traditional alcohol biomarkers include gamma glutamyltransferase (GGT), aspartate aminotransferase (AST), alanine aminotransferase (ALT), and mean corpuscular volume (MCV). Elevations in GGT, AST and ALT have been associated with heavy alcohol use. An elevated GGT is not a very sensitive biomarker and is only elevated in about 30 to 50 percent of heavy drinkers. AST and ALT are less sensitive measures of alcohol dependence than GGT [18]. Furthermore, the AST and ALT are even less accurate biomarkers in patients under age 30 and over age 70 [18]. An increase in MCV has been associated with chronic heavy drinking but only has a sensitivity of about 47 percent and is not specific to heavy alcohol use [18]. In addition, the MCV can stay elevated for several months after one discontinues alcohol use.

Serum carbohydrate-deficient transferrin (CDT) is a more useful biomarker in identifying alcohol dependence and in monitoring drinking behavior because CDT serum elevations and declines occur relatively quickly with the onset and termination of alcohol consumption. Heavy drinking (greater than 60 grams of alcohol per day - 4 to 5 standard drinks/day) for a period of 2 weeks will usually cause elevation in the CDT [18]. With abstinence serum level of CDT drops within 2 weeks which is quicker than GGT. Therefore CDT can be a better predictor of relapse and remission. Serum CDT has greater sensitivity (up to 83 percent) and specificity (up to 92 percent) than the GGT, AST, ALT and MCV. Researchers are currently looking for more accurate biomarkers to help clinicians identify, treat and monitor alcohol use disorders [18].

Lastly, one can monitor individuals for alcohol use with one of the continuous alcohol monitoring ankle bracelets used frequently by law enforcement and court ordered treatment programs.

Non-Pharmacologic Interventions

Alcohol Anonymous (AA) 12 step programs are most common and studies have shown that medication management programs are also effective. Individualized treatment is recommended. Please see the section on non-pharmacologic treatments for substance use disorders in Chapter one for more information.

Pathophysiology of Alcohol Use Disorders (AUD)

Research indicates that alcohol use disorders are psychiatric diagnoses associated with underlying neurochemical changes. This research strongly supports the concept that addiction to alcohol is truly a chronic medical disease like diabetes responsive to pharmacologic interventions.

Multiple neurotransmitters are involved in the development of AUDs, including glutamate (GLU), gamma-aminobutyric acid (GABA), endogenous opioids, dopamine (DA), serotonin (5-HT), corticotrophin releasing factor (CRF), and neuropeptide Y (NPY). Acutely alcohol enhances GABA transmission through the GABA-A receptor, decreases glutaminergic transmission through inhibition of the N-methyl-D-aspartic acid (NDMA) receptors and facilitates dopaminergic, opioidergic, serotonergic, noradrenergic, and endocannabinoid signaling [19].

It is the activation of mesolimbic and mesocortical dopaminergic pathways that mediates the acute positive reinforcing properties of alcohol. Neurobiologic changes that occur later are thought to mediate the negative reinforcing effects of heavy chronic alcohol use.

Medications play a strong role in the treatment of medical illnesses without bias, but for some, the treatment of alcohol based illnesses with medications is hard to accept. Cognitive and behavioral processes along with life style changes are cornerstones of the treatment of all mental health and medical conditions including the treatment of AUDs.

Treatment of AUDs needs to be individualized and experience indicates psychosocial, group and individual psychotherapy, as well as psychopharmacological treatments can be successful treatments alone or as combination therapy. As in medical disorders treatment non-adherence greatly affects the outcome of these therapies.

Another major factor affecting the success of medications in the treatment of AUD is the individual's alcoholic subtype or genetic makeup. Several studies looking at alcohol dependence [20] have demonstrated that individuals with Type B alcohol dependence (early onset/more severe) respond preferentially to treatments *versus* those with Type A (late onset/less severe). Genetic variables, such as the Asn40Asp40 heterozygote *versus* Anp40Anp40 homozygote receptor variation, also may predict medication response.

Reward drinking appears to be mediated *via* mesolimbic dopaminergic activation. Mesolimbic activation is associated with motivation and plays a role in regulation of our response to natural reinforcers (food, sex, social interaction). Dopaminergic firing in the mesolimbic region leads to increased DA firing in the ventral tegmental area of the midbrain with resulting increases of DA action in the nucleus accumbens (NA) (ventral striatum) and other regions of the limbic forebrain. Alcohol also activates this pathway in an indirect way by means of activating beta-endorphins that innervate the ventral tegmental area and the nucleus accumbens resulting in activation/excitation of the NA. Medications that antagonize this pathway may decrease the reward aspect of alcohol use leading to a decrease in drinking. Agents of interest would be antagonists of dopamine, GABA, 5HT3 serotonin and/or opioid receptors [21].

PHARMACOTHERAPY FOR ALCOHOL USE DISORDERS (AUD)

Management of Outpatient Alcohol Withdrawal

Patient assessment needs to include comorbid medical conditions and medications, a careful history of alcohol use, amount and duration of use, past attempts to quit and any previous withdrawal seizures or delirium tremens. An alcohol blood level can be a determining factor in managing withdrawal as an outpatient or an inpatient. Motivation for sobriety can be important in assessing the likelihood a patient would drink on the medication used to manage the withdrawal.

Traditional management of outpatient alcohol withdrawal has involved the use of a long acting benzodiazepine such as chlordiazepoxide. Shorter acting agents such as lorazepam and oxazepam can also be used but provide a shorter duration of coverage. Benzodiazepines are still considered the gold standard management, however other medication alternatives are available and medication selection needs to be individualized [22 - 25].

Of concern with the benzodiazepines is the potential that the patient may drink on top of this treatment. Alcohol in combination with benzodiazepines can be a deadly combination. In these individuals an anticonvulsant medication such as valproic acid or gabapentin may be preferred because of minimal risk for adverse/lethal events when combine with alcohol use.

Supplemental medications may be needed to manage associated symptoms like nausea, pain and insomnia. Vitamin therapy with thiamine, folate and a multivitamin given daily is recommended because malnutrition and vitamin deficiency is common with alcoholism and supplementation can help treat and prevent serious neurological conditions related to alcoholism.

Table 2. Management of outpatient alcohol withdrawal.

Agent	Dosing	Concerns
Benzodiazepines – FDA approved		
Chlordiazepoxide (Librium)	3-day supply 50–100 mg every 6 hours for 4 doses, then 25–50 mg every 6 hours for 8 doses Dose depends on degree of withdrawal	Specific dosing directions should be given to the patient Caution in combination with alcohol Adequate liver function is required
Lorazepam (Ativan)	2–4 mg every 6 hours for 4 doses, then 1–2 mg every 6 hours for 8 doses	Not metabolized No active metabolites Good if liver dysfunction is present Caution in combination with alcohol
Anticonvulsants - Non-FDA Approved *		
Valproic Acid (Depakote, Depakene)	5 day supply - 500 mg 4 times on day 1 500 mg 3 times on day 2 500 mg 2 times on day 3 500 mg HS on days 4 and 5	Adequate liver function is required, not if pregnant or current / history of pancreatitis Minimal risk when used with alcohol
Gabapentin (Neurontin)	600mg 3 times a day on days 1-3 300mg 3 times a day on day 4 300mg 2 times a day on day 5 300mg a day on day 6	Renal elimination Minimal risk when used with alcohol

* Can consider topiramate (25) and carbamazepine (22)
Adapted from references [22 - 24]

FDA Approved Medications for Alcohol Use Disorder [26]

Since the early fifties only four products have been approved by the Federal Drug Administration (FDA) for the treatment of alcohol dependence (AD) - disulfiram, naltrexone oral (PO) and long-acting intramuscular (IM) formulations and acamprosate.

Research has demonstrated that these medications are not identical in their effects on alcohol dependence, targeting different aspects of craving, protracted withdrawal symptoms, relapse and abstinence. There is a growing wealth of data supporting the idea that they each target different subtypes of patients with AD.

There have been several reviews of the research on these agents supporting their roles in the treatment of AD. More recent research has been focused on the efficacy of combination therapies, use of non-FDA approved agents, targeting additional neurochemicals and pathways involved in alcohol dependence and attempting to identify patient variables that might predict response to treatment [21, 27 - 29].

Disulfiram (Antabuse®) [19, 21, 27]

Approved in 1951, disulfiram is the oldest medication treatment for AD and is a form of aversive therapy. The goal of disulfiram use is to assist the patient in maintaining abstinence from alcohol thereby avoiding the negative consequences of drinking while taking disulfiram.

Disulfiram works by irreversibly inhibiting the enzyme acetaldehyde dehydrogenase resulting in elevated levels of acetaldehyde in the blood stream when alcohol is ingested. These higher levels result in the “disulfiram reaction”. The disulfiram reaction can range from mild to life threatening depending on the amount of alcohol consumed and can last from half an hour to several hours. Symptoms include flushing, nausea, vomiting, severe headache, dizziness, blurred vision, chest pain, shortness of breath, hyperventilation, tachycardia, hypotension, syncope and confusion. In more severe cases the reaction may result in cardiac arrhythmias, respiratory depression, cardiovascular collapse, seizures, loss of consciousness and death.

The rates of non-adherence with disulfiram therapy are high and contribute to its low success rate. Best used in a highly motivated individual and given where medication dosing can be observed. Disulfiram appears to decrease the number of drinking days but has no effect on craving for alcohol, nor does it appear to promote ongoing abstinence, its primary effect is as a psychological deterrent to drinking. But many AD patients will drink even on disulfiram.

Naltrexone (Revia® (PO), Vivitrol® (IM))

Naltrexone was the second agent approved by the FDA for the treatment of alcohol dependence. A once daily oral tablet formulation was approved in 1994, followed by the once monthly intramuscular depot injection in 2006.

Naltrexone is an opioid receptor antagonist with primary activity at the mu opiate receptor. Alcohol use triggers the release of endogenous opioid peptides that results in dopamine release in the mesolimbic area, contributing to the positive reinforcing effects of alcohol use. Naltrexone blocks alcohol induced euphoria, mitigates craving, decreases overall alcohol intake and number of drinking days, decreases relapse rates, and increases days abstinent. Naltrexone appears to decrease the positive reinforcement associated with alcohol use enabling the alcoholic that does drink to get back to sobriety more readily. It may also be effective in decreasing the severity of alcohol related problems [21]. Naltrexone's ability to block the positive reinforcing effects of alcohol has been demonstrated to assist in decreasing craving in Type II alcoholics in which reward craving is characteristic [28].

Adherence to treatment has a major effect on the success rate of naltrexone therapy for alcohol dependence. This is complicated by the desire to use alcohol. Use of the depot formulation may assist with adherence and success of therapy [29]. In conjunction with cognitive behavioral treatment naltrexone on the short term appears to decrease relapse and increased retention in treatment programs, while mid-term use decreases craving and increases the time to the first drink. Naltrexone therapy is continued even if the patient drinks, the goal is to minimize the relapse and get them back into treatment.

Prior to initiating naltrexone therapy a naloxone challenge test or a urine drug screen test for opioids/opiates is suggested. A positive test would indicate the need for opioid/opiate detoxification prior to starting naltrexone in order to prevent acute opioid/opiate withdrawal. Patient's with comorbid opioid/opiate use disorders will need to be educated that naltrexone will decrease the patient's tolerance to previous doses of narcotics, and if used to "over-ride" the blockade in an attempt to get high can result in life-threatening overdose or death.

Patients requiring narcotics for chronic pain would not be candidates for naltrexone. In situations requiring the emergent acute use of opioid analgesics, higher doses will be required and close monitoring will be necessary. Discontinuation of naltrexone prior to elective surgery is necessary.

Table 3. Dosing of disulfiram, naltrexone and acamprosate.

Medication	Dosing (mg/day)	Side Effects/Cautions/Interactions	Information
Antabuse (Disulfiram®)	Initial dose: 250mg increasing to 500mg in 1-2 weeks Maintenance Doses: 125-500mg/day	Side Effects: Halitosis Dysgeusia: metallic or garlic-like taste Cautions: Diabetes, brain damage, hypothyroidism, renal and hepatic disease or epilepsy. Contraindications: severe myocardial disease and coronary occlusion. Drug Interactions: Alcohol, metronidazole, omeprazole, paraldehyde; caution with alcohol containing cold/allergy preparations, mouthwash, hand cleansers	First dose is given at least 12 hours after the last drink Duration of effect is roughly 1-2 weeks after medication discontinuation as new enzyme is synthesized Pregnancy Category: B Lactation: Infant risk cannot be ruled out
Naltrexone (Revia®) (Vivitrol®)	PO: Initial: 12.5-25mg Increasing every 3 days Maintenance: 50-100mg LA-IM: 380mg every 4 weeks Deep IM gluteal injection alternating gluteal muscles each injection. Only use the needles and diluents provided	PO Side Effects: Nausea, diarrhea, loss of appetite, headache, arthralgia, dizziness, anxiety, depression, constipation, flu-like syndrome, and upper-respiratory tract infection. LA-IM: Injection site pain, swelling, tenderness, bruising, rash, or redness. Caution: Opiate use, hepatic disease Contraindications: Acute hepatitis, liver failure. Need for chronic narcotics for pain. Black Box Warning: Hepatocellular injury when given in excessive oral doses (5x normal)	Side effects are due to the medication itself not an interaction with alcohol. Use of the depot formulation may minimize side effects due to dosing peak blood levels and may decrease the likelihood of hepatic toxicity. Pregnancy Category: C Lactation: Infant risk cannot be ruled out

(Table 3) contd.....

Medication	Dosing (mg/day)	Side Effects/Cautions/Interactions	Information
Acamprosate (Campral®)	Initial: 333-666mg three times a day with meals Therapeutic dose is 666mg/day	Side Effects: Diarrhea, vomiting, abdominal pain, nausea, decreased appetite, anxiety, depression, insomnia, dry mouth, dizziness, gas, paresthesia, somnolence Cautions: Contraindicated in severe renal disease	Initiated after withdrawal has resolved Adherence can be affected by TID dosing Dose is decreased in renal disease Pregnancy Category: C Lactation Rating: Infant risk cannot be ruled out.

Adapted from references [20, 21, 28 - 30]

Acamprosate (Campral®) [21, 28, 30]

The most recent FDA approved agent for alcohol dependence is acamprosate, used in Europe for years prior to this, acamprosate was approved in the United States in 2004. Acamprosate is indicated for maintaining abstinence in patients who have achieved abstinence and as part of a comprehensive treatment program.

Acamprosate is a glutaminergic antagonist, acamprosate is thought to have its primary action at the metabotropic NMDA receptors. The chronic progression of intoxication and withdrawal is believed to result in a hyperglutaminergic state in the Central Nervous System (CNS). Acamprosate appears to block this development and decreases dependence induced drinking. Because acamprosate also has GABAergic activity it is thought to normalize the GABA and glutaminergic systems resulting in decreased alcohol dependence. Because of the above mechanisms acamprosate may target relief drinking. Acamprosate may extend the time before relapse and decrease alcohol intake. Motivation for abstinence may be a key factor in success of treatment with acamprosate.

Therapy with acamprosate is continued even if the patient drinks, the goal is to minimize the relapse and get the patient back into treatment.

Combination Therapy

Because naltrexone and acamprosate have different mechanism of actions, it would be logical to believe that the combination of these agents would result in even better treatment outcomes. A European study on the combination of naltrexone and acamprosate *versus* each agent alone and placebo demonstrated this additive benefit. With the combination demonstrating superiority to naltrexone alone which was superior to acamprosate and all three treatment groups were better than placebo [31]. On the other hand, the US NIAAA COMBINE trial did not support the use of the combination of naltrexone and acamprosate over naltrexone alone in measures of percent days abstinent and time to first heavy drinking day. The study also failed to show effectiveness for acamprosate while demonstrating that naltrexone significantly decreased heavy drinking days [27].

In a subset of the COMBINE trial that looked at the response of individuals with Type A *versus* Type B AD to naltrexone or placebo in combination with Medication Management (MM) alone or MM in combination with Combined Behavioral Intervention (CBI), it was demonstrated that Type A alcoholics responded to naltrexone but those with Type B did not. Further, in those individuals treated with naltrexone and MM benefit was limited to the group with Type A AD. There were no significant effects seen with CBI in either group [32].

Although European and American studies are not in agreement on the efficacy of the combination or acamprosate there appears to be a study paradigm difference in the patient populations used in these studies. Patients in the European trials had an increased severity and were more commonly in inpatient detoxification programs which may indicate a patient subtype that may respond better to acamprosate than others.

A more recent combination trial studied the combination of disulfiram and acamprosate. The combination group in this open label study had a longer period of abstinence than either drug or placebo alone [20].

Non-FDA Approved Pharmacotherapies for AD

Lack of response or intolerance to the FDA approved medications for alcohol use disorder has driven research to non-approved agents to treat substance use disorders. Several agents showing potential include memantine, baclofen, topiramate, gabapentin, ondansetron, and the selective serotonergic reuptake inhibitor antidepressants.

SUMMARY

Alcohol use disorders are chronic illnesses with a remitting and relapsing course. The development of an AUD has many roots and is expressed in a variety of different ways. Being able to recognize an individual with an issue with alcohol is the first step. Assisting the individual with an AUD in maintaining sobriety will take a unique individualized treatment approach that includes appropriate cognitive and behavioral interventions, lifestyle changes and medication management. It is also imperative to address co-morbid conditions and lingering issues such as insomnia.

CLINICAL VIGNETTE RESOLUTION

Karen has been sober for the past year with the help of acamprosate therapy and has reconciled with her husband. They are now planning a family and she wants to know if acamprosate is safe to continue during pregnancy.

Pregnancy ratings for the different medication options are category B for disulfiram, and category C for naltrexone and acamprosate. Infant risk could still be involved even if she were to switch to disulfiram. The question would be whether or not disulfiram is less problematic than drinking while pregnant. Alternatively, a trial of SSRI antidepressant therapy could be prescribed, but the data for these agents in maintaining sobriety is not as robust as the FDA approved medications. These medications have their own concerns in pregnancy.

After conferring with her husband and obstetrician, Karen decides to stop acamprosate and start disulfiram 250mg daily.

PROVIDER RESOURCES

National Institute on Alcohol Abuse and Alcoholism http://www.niaaa.nih.gov/

National Council on Alcoholism and Drug Dependence, Inc.
http://www.ncadd.org/

ALCOHOL USE DISORDERS: PATIENT EDUCATION SHEET

Alcohal Use Disorders (AUDS)?

AUDs are characterized by a pattern of drinking excessively despite the negative effects of alcohol on your work, family, educational and social activities. Use continues even when faced with medical and legal issues. AUDs involve a number of symptoms including tolerance to or withdrawal from alcohol, using more alcohol at a time than planned and/or for a longer time than planned. It may also involve having trouble reducing the use of alcohol. Indications of a problem with alcohol include drinking alone, to escape problems, or just to get drunk; hiding alcohol about the home; getting irritated when you are unable to obtain alcohol to drink and avoiding activities that do not involve drinking.

Questions to ask yourself if you are concerned about your use of alcohol:

1. Have you ever felt you should cut down on your drinking?
2. Have people annoyed you by criticizing your drinking?
3. Have you ever felt bad or guilty about your drinking?
4. Have you ever had a drink first thing in the morning to steady your nerves or get rid of a hangover (eye-opener)?

Two "yes" answers to the above questions indicates a possible alcohol problem that you should discuss with your doctor. (acponline.org accessed 7/26/13)

Are AUDs Common?

Alcohol abuse affects about 10% of women and 20% of men in the United States.

What are the Signs of Alcohol Intoxication?

Early use may result in disinhibition, a feeling of wellbeing, more relaxed, social and outgoing. A person may do or say things that they would normally not do. As the blood alcohol level rises alcohol becomes a depressant and can cause confusion, emotional liability, concentration problems, motor impairment and over sedation.

What are the Signs of Alcohol Withdrawal?

As the blood level of alcohol in our body drops you can experience withdrawal symptoms: trembling or the shakes; irritability, anxiety or jumpiness; sweating, nausea and vomiting, insomnia, depression, fatigue or loss of appetite and headaches. Severe withdrawal from alcohol can be life-threatening. Sometimes called delirium tremens or the "DTs" and involves the general withdrawal symptoms with the addition of hallucinations, confusion, seizures, fever, and severe agitation. Severe withdrawal or the DTs is an emergency situation and needs to be treated in a hospital.

Is Alcohol Addictive?

Yes.

What are the Complications of Alcohol Use?

Chronic use of alcohol can damage your liver, heart, brain, pancreas and immune system. It can also result in the development of cancer.

How are Alcohol Use Disorders Diagnosed?

Doctors diagnose an alcohol use disorder, generally known as alcohol abuse or alcoholism, when a patient's drinking causes distress or harm.

What are the Treatment Options?

There are many treatments options for alcohol use disorders and treatment should be individualized. While some people with alcohol dependence can cut back or stop drinking without help, most are only able to do so temporarily unless they get treatment.

Non-medication Options: individual and group counseling, support groups (*i.e.*, Alcoholics Anonymous), residential treatment, medications, drug testing, and/or relapse-prevention programs.

Medication Options: Medications can help us avoid using alcohol and decrease the craving for alcohol. They work best when combined with non-drug therapies.

These medications include: Antabuse, Revia, Campral. Ask your provider if one of these may be right for you.

PATIENT RESOURCES

Websites

HelpGuide.Org is an online resource on many Mental Health Issues. They provide education on the disease state and treatment and links to other resources. http://www.helpguide.org/mental/alcohol_abuse_alcoholism_signs_effects_treatment.htm

National Institute on Alcohol Abuse and Alcoholism
http://www.niaaa.nih.gov/

National Council on Alcoholism and Drug Dependence, Inc.
http://www.ncadd.org/

Online Articles

Medicine Net "Alcohol Abuse and Alcoholism"
http://www.medicinenet.com/alcohol_abuse_and_alcoholism/article.htm

Mayo Clinic "Alcoholism"
http://www.mayoclinic.com/health/alcoholism/DS00340

WebMD Understanding Alcohol Abuse and Treatment
http://www.webmd.com/mental-health/alcohol-abuse/understanding-alcohol-abuse-treatment

CONFLICT OF INTEREST

The authors confirm that they have no conflict of interest to declare for this publication.

ACKNOWLEDGEMENTS

Declared none.

REFERENCES

[1] Updating Estimates of the Economic Costs of Alcohol Abuse in the United States: Estimates, Update Methods, and Data Report prepared by The Lewin Group for the National Institute on Alcohol Abuse and Alcoholism. Rockville, MD: NIAAA, National Institutes of Health, Department of Health and Human Services 2000.

[2] Mannelli P, Pae CU. Medical comorbidity and alcohol dependence. Curr Psychiatry Rep 2007; 9(3): 217-24.
[http://dx.doi.org/10.1007/s11920-007-0022-x] [PMID: 17521518]

[3] Walker RD, Howard MO, Lambert MD, Suchinsky R. Psychiatric and medical comorbidities of veterans with substance use disorders. Hosp Community Psychiatry 1994; 45(3): 232-7.
[PMID: 8188193]

[4] National Council on Alcoholism and Drug Dependence. Alcoholism and alcohol-related problems: a sobering look. NCADD Fact Sheet. Available online: ncadd.org

[5] US Department of Health and Human Services (DHHS). Tenth Special Report to Congress on Alcohol and Health. Bethesda, MD: DHHS; 2000. Available from: pubs.niaaa.nih.gov/publications/10report/intro.pdf , [cited: 28th August 2006];

[6] Mokdad AH, Marks JS, Stroup DF, Gerberding JL. Actual causes of death in the United States, 2000. JAMA 2004; 291(10): 1238-45.
[http://dx.doi.org/10.1001/jama.291.10.1238] [PMID: 15010446]

[7] Grant BF, Dawson DA, Stinson FS, Chou SP, Dufour MC, Pickering RP. The 12-month prevalence and trends in DSM-IV alcohol abuse and dependence: United States, 1991-1992 and 2001-2002. Drug Alcohol Depend 2004; 74(3): 223-34.
[http://dx.doi.org/10.1016/j.drugalcdep.2004.02.004] [PMID: 15194200]

[8] Johnston LD, O'Malley PM, Bachman JG, Schulenberg JE. Various stimulant drugs show continuing gradual declines among teens in 2008, most illicit drugs hold steady. Ann Arbor, MI: University of Michigan News Service 2008.

[9] Age of Drinking Onset Predicts Future Alcohol Abuse and Dependence Jan 14, 1998. The analysis by Grant BF and Dawson DA. NIAAA's Division of Biometry and Epidemiology, is published in the January issue of the Journal of Substance Abuse and based on the NIAAA-sponsored National Longitudinal Alcohol Epidemiologic Survey (NLAES). www.niaaa.nih.gov/NewsEvents/NewsReleases/aging.htm

[10] Reich T, Edenberg HJ, Goate A, *et al.* Genome-wide search for genes affecting the risk for alcohol dependence. Am J Med Genet 1998; 81(3): 207-15. [Neuropsychiatr Genet].
[http://dx.doi.org/10.1002/(SICI)1096-8628(19980508)81:3<207::AID-AJMG1>3.0.CO;2-T] [PMID: 9603606]

[11] Heath AC, Bucholz KK, Madden PA, *et al.* Genetic and environmental contributions to alcohol dependence risk in a national twin sample: consistency of findings in women and men. Psychol Med 1997; 27(6): 1381-96.
[http://dx.doi.org/10.1017/S0033291797005643] [PMID: 9403910]

[12] Prescott CA, Kendler KS. Genetic and environmental contributions to alcohol abuse and dependence

in a population-based sample of male twins. Am J Psychiatry 1999; 156(1): 34-40. [http://dx.doi.org/10.1176/ajp.156.1.34] [PMID: 9892295]

[13] Goodwin DW, Schulsinger F, Hermansen L, Guze SB, Winokur G. Alcohol problems in adoptees raised apart from alcoholic biological parents. Arch Gen Psychiatry 1973; 28(2): 238-43. [http://dx.doi.org/10.1001/archpsyc.1973.01750320068011] [PMID: 4684290]

[14] O'Brien CP. The CAGE questionnaire for detection of alcoholism: a remarkably useful but simple tool. JAMA 2008; 300(17): 2054-6. [http://dx.doi.org/10.1001/jama.2008.570] [PMID: 18984895]

[15] Williams RR, Horm JW. Association of cancer sites with tobacco and alcohol consumption and socioeconomic status of patients: interview study from the Third National Cancer Survey. J Natl Cancer Inst 1977; 58(3): 525-47. [PMID: 557114]

[16] Genkinger JM, Spiegelman D, Anderson KE, *et al.* Alcohol intake and pancreatic cancer risk: a pooled analysis of fourteen cohort studies. Cancer Epidemiol Biomarkers Prev 2009; 18(3): 765-76. [http://dx.doi.org/10.1158/1055-9965.EPI-08-0880] [PMID: 19258474]

[17] William J. Alcohol and Cancer. Cancer Research. American Association for Cancer Research 1992; 52: 2119-23.

[18] Peterson K. Biomarkers for alcohol use and abuse-a summary. Alcohol Res. Health. Available from: http://pubs.niaaa.nih.gov/publications/arh28-1/30-37.pdf 2004-2005; 28(1): 30-7. [PMID: 19006989]

[19] Diagnostic and Statistical Manual of Mental Disorders. 4th ed., Washington, D.C.: American Psychiatric Association 1994.

[20] Garbutt JC. The state of pharmacotherapy for the treatment of alcohol dependence. J Subst Abuse Treat 2009; 36(1): S15-23. [PMID: 19062347]

[21] Swift R. Emerging approaches to managing alcohol dependence. Am J Health-Syst Pharm 2007; 64 (Suppl 3): 12-22. [http://dx.doi.org/10.2146/ajhp060644]

[22] Modesto-Lowe V, Huard J, Conrad C. Alcohol withdrawal kindling: is there a role for anticonvulsants? Psychiatry (Edgmont) 2005; 2(5): 25-31. [PMID: 21152146]

[23] Spiegel DR, Radac D. Alcohol withdrawal when to choose an adjunctive anticonvulsant. Curr Psychiatr 2010; 9(4): 27-39.

[24] Stock CJ, Carpenter L, Ying J, Greene T. Gabapentin *versus* chlordiazepoxide for outpatient alcohol detoxification treatment. Ann Pharmacother 2013; 47(7-8): 961-9.

[25] Kenna GA, Lomastro TL, Schiesl A, Leggio L, Swift RM. Review of topiramate: an antiepileptic for the treatment of alcohol dependence. Curr Drug Abuse Rev 2009; 2(2): 135-42. [http://dx.doi.org/10.2174/1874473710902020135] [PMID: 19630744]

[26] Diagnostic and Statistical Manual of Mental Disorders. 5th ed., Arlington, VA: American Psychiatric Association 2013.

[27] Johnson BA. Update on neuropharmacological treatments for alcoholism: scientific basis and clinical findings. Biochem Pharmacol 2008; 75(1): 34-56.
[http://dx.doi.org/10.1016/j.bcp.2007.08.005] [PMID: 17880925]

[28] Heilig M, Egli M. Pharmacological treatment of alcohol dependence: target symptoms and target mechanisms. Pharmacol Ther 2006; 111(3): 855-76.
[http://dx.doi.org/10.1016/j.pharmthera.2006.02.001] [PMID: 16545872]

[29] Garbutt JC, Kranzler HR, O'Malley SS, *et al.* Efficacy and tolerability of long-acting injectable naltrexone for alcohol dependence: a randomized controlled trial. JAMA 2005; 293(13): 1617-25.
[http://dx.doi.org/10.1001/jama.293.13.1617] [PMID: 15811981]

[30] Kenna GA, McGeary JE, Swift RM. Pharmacotherapy, pharmacogenomics and the future of treatment for alcohol dependence, part 2. Am J Health Syst Pharm 2004; 61: 2380-90.
[PMID: 15581261]

[31] Tolliver BK, McRae A, Sonne SC, Brady KT. Safety and tolerability of acamprosate in alcohol-dependent individuals with bipolar disorder. Addict Disord Their Treat 2009; 8: 33-8.
[http://dx.doi.org/10.1097/ADT.0b013e31816719df]

[32] Kiefer F, Jahn H, Tarnaske T, *et al.* Comparing and combining naltrexone and acamprosate in relapse prevention of alcoholism: a double-blind, placebo-controlled study. Arch Gen Psychiatry 2003; 60(1): 92-9.
[http://dx.doi.org/10.1001/archpsyc.60.1.92] [PMID: 12511176]

[33] Anton RF, O'Malley SS, Ciraulo DA, *et al.* Combined pharmacotherapies and behavioral interventions for alcohol dependence: the COMBINE study: a randomized controlled trial. JAMA 2006; 295(17): 2003-17.
[http://dx.doi.org/10.1001/jama.295.17.2003] [PMID: 16670409]

CHAPTER 8

Anabolic-Androgenic Steroids (AAS) Related Disorders

Aly Hassan[1,*], **Subhash C. Bhatia**[2,3] and **Shashi K. Bhatia**[4]

[1] *Phoenix VA Health Care System, Department of Psychiatry, University of Arizona, Phoenix College of Medicine, Gilbert VA Clinic, 3285 S Val Vista Drive, Gilbert AZ 85925, USA*

[2] *Department of Psychiatry, Mental Health and Behavioral Sciences, Creighton University*

[3] *Department VA Nebraska- Western Iowa Health Care System 4101 Woolworth Ave Omaha, NE 68105, USA*

[4] *Departments of Psychiatry and Pediatrics, Division of Child and Adolescent Psychiatry, Creighton University, 3528 Dodge Omaha, NE 68131, USA*

Abstract: This chapter discusses epidemiologic, pathophysiology and diagnostic issues associated with long term none medical use of Anabolic Androgenic Steroids (AAS) .These agents are synthetic derivatives of the hormone testosterone with higher bioavailability and activity [1]. These drugs are used by athletes to gain muscle mass thereby gaining advantage. As a result many users often don't disclose their use to their doctors [2, 3]. Medical complications may include, hypertension, cardiomyopathy and hypogonadism. Psychiatric complications may include mood and psychotic disorders [4]. Withdrawal may lead to dysphoria and irritability. Patients usually do not consider themselves as addicted. They traditionally think that they are more knowledgeable about these drugs than their doctors [2, 3]. In USA, AAS are currently schedule class III drugs requiring prescription, however they can be easily obtained online from other countries.

KEY LEARNING POINTS

1. Illicit Anabolic steroid none medical use poses a worldwide public health problem.

* **Corresponding author Aly Hassan:** Phoenix VA Health Care System, Associate Clinical Professor of Psychiatry, University of Arizona, Phoenix College of Medicine, USA; Tel: 480-825-7225, 402-714-1188; Email: Aly.hassan@va.gov

2. About 30% of Anabolic steroid users develop a clinical dependence syndrome with, chronic use despite adverse effects on physical, psychosocial, occupational or school functioning [5].
3. Dozens of formulations exist with different administrations routs (oral, IM and IV injection, and topically in the form of cream or gel. Amounts used may reach 10 to 100 times the usual therapeutic doses.
4. Medical morbidity with AAS use may include hypertension, dyslipidemia, cardiomyopathy, hypogonadism, hepatic dysfunction and HIV/AIDS hepatitis B and C due to sharing dirty needles.
5. AAS have been associated with the development of mania, hypomania, psychosis or uncontrolled anger ("roid rage"). AAS withdrawal symptoms are associated with craving, irritability, dysphoria, depression with or without suicidality.
6. AAS differ from classical drugs in that intoxication produce little immediate reward or "high", but instead has a delayed reward of muscle mass gain or "bulking".
7. Anabolic Steroids are classified in Schedule III. Among all the substances in Schedules II or III ASS are the only ones that are no identified with a specific use disorder in DSM- 5 [5].
8. AAS are illegal in the USA without a medical Prescription, But they are available over the counter in many countries, and are easily ordered online.
9. Anabolic steroid use can be a gateway drug to other substances including opioids [6].

CLINICAL VIGNETTE

A 17 year old male presented with his mother for a follow up appointment with his pediatrician. The lab results showed high LDL and low HDL, mild elevations of AST and ALT. blood pressure was 132/89. The initial reason for the visit was the treatment of acne on the upper back and chest that was resistant to over the counter treatment. The patient stated that he was currently a member of the high school football team, and that he had gained significant weight in the previous year. His mother complained that his gets easily angered, On one occasion she asked him to leave the house until he calms down. She noted that patient spent more time in the gym, He spends much less time with with his girlfriend or playing his guitar with his friends as he used to do. His grades were falling and he was skipping school in order to go to the gym .

EPIDEMIOLOGY

Epidemiological survey in the US in the last 2 decades have estimated that 3% to 11% of male high school students have used AAS. The number of AAS users in the United States is estimated around 3 millions [7].

Anabolic steroid users are mostly none athletes who use the drugs for cosmetic reasons. A subset of this group suffers from an excessive a preoccupation by body image muscle dysmorphia (a subjective perception of being small and week) [8],

Research pointed out that Up to 6% of athletes abuse anabolic steroids to enhance performance in competitive sports or just a desire to increase physical attractiveness [7]. The 2004 Monitoring the Future report noted that that there was a decline in use among adolescents in grades 8 and 10 but not among 12th graders.

About 30% of anabolic-androgenic steroids users appear to develop the classical picture of dependence syndrome.

2.7-2.9% of young American adults have taken AAS at least once in their lives [9].

DIAGNOSIS, AND CLINICAL PRESENTATION

DSM-5 does not have specific anabolic-androgenic steroid use disorder listed. However the symptoms and signs of these disorders can fit in the in one or more of the following categories.

Other (or unknown) Substance–Related Disorders, Other (or unknown) Substance Use Disorder, Other (unknown) Substance Withdrawal, Other (or unknown) Substance– Induced Disorders or Unspecified Other (or unknown) Substance–Related Disorder (non-substance use) disorder".

Individuals using ASS may present with well-developed muscularity of the upper body with on occasions needle marks in large muscles, acne, pigmented striae on skin, excessive facial body hair, obsession with weight training, dissatisfaction with appearance, sense of invincibility and grandiosity .

ASS have a he wide range of Physical and psychiatric effects and adverse effects, the fact that Steroid receptors are present in nearly all cell types, explain why organ system is affected by anabolic steroids.

1. Endocrine effects: In men causes infertility, breast development, decreased endogenous testosterone, shrinking of testicles, male pattern of baldness and prostate enlargement. In women causes enlargement of clitoris, excessive body hair, voice deepening and male pattern of baldness.
2. Musculoskeletal system: short stature in adolescents, increased muscle mass and higher risk of tendon injuries.
3. Cardiovascular system: Increased LDL, decreased HDL, risk of atherosclerosis, hypertension, coronary artery disease, cardiomyopathy and polycythemia.
4. Liver: Enlargement, cancer, peliosis hepatic cysts and tumors.
5. Skin: Acne and cysts, oily scalp, jaundice, fluid retention.
6. Metabolic: Glucose intolerance.
7. Infections: HIV/AIDS and hepatitis B and C due to needle sharing.
8. Psychiatric: Rage, aggression ("roid rage"), mania, psychosis, delusions and depression with or without suicidality Treatment [8].

PHYSIOLOGY AND PHARMACOLOGY

Testosterone is produced in the body from cholesterol. .In men Testicles produce most of the hormone, while adrenal glands only play a secondary role. In females, testosterone is produced in the adrenal glands and the ovaries. Normal total plasma testosterone level in males varies between 300 -1,000 ng/dl. Most of the hormone is bound to protein and is inactive; free testosterone, is the active form and only 2% to 3% of the total levels .

Testosterone is metabolized into 1) dihydrotestosterone, which has several folds more potency than testosterone, and 2) estradiol, which has feminizing effects. Testosterone is inactive when taken orally and is rapidly inactivated by the liver when injected.

Dozens of Anabolic steroids formulations are available. Some are designed with the goal of limiting the potential side effects while others were designed specifically to reduce the potential of detection by antidoping means.

Commonly abused anabolic steroids include: oxymetholone (Anadrol), oxadrolone (Oxadrin), methaandrostenolone (Dianabol), stanozolol (Winstrol), fluoxymesterone (Halotestin) and nandrolone (such as Durabolin) nandrolone decanoate (Deca-Durabolin), testosterone cypionate (Depo-Testostrerone).

Steroid users tend to use these agents in patterns (Cycles) to minimize side effects and maximize muscle gain, Cycling consists of taking using a specific anabolic steroid over a period of time alternating with periods of interruption. Stacking is the practice of combining different anabolic agents generally through different routes of administration. Pyramiding is the gradual increase of the dose and frequency of one or more agents to reach a peak dose followed by a gradual reduction of the dose until discontinuation, with cycles lasting in general between 6-12 weeks.

BIO-PSYCHO-SOCIAL TREATMENT

Pharmacological Treatment of Anabolic Steroids Disorders

Pharmacotherapy is of only adjunctive value, it is limited to addressing Endocrine (to restore functioning of the hypothalamic-pituitary-gonadal axis), physical and psychiatric symptoms. Medications for psychiatric symptoms should be based on balancing the pros and cons, including their potential side-effects. Depression is common during AAS withdrawal. Antidepressants are indicated when symptoms of depression persist. Selective serotonin reuptake inhibitors (SSRIs) such as fluoxetine are effective both for depression and dysmorphic symptoms. Antipsychotic drugs may be needed to treat persistent and marked irritability, agitation or psychosis. To withdraw steroids, it is reasonable to taper off high doses gradually [10].

Clonidine (Catapres) may help in addressing symptoms of withdrawals, as some researchers postulate an opiate-like withdrawal mechanism.

Psycho-Social Interventions

Supportive therapy is the main stay of treatment,. Initiatives to educate high risk groups (high school football players and the in reducing and preventing) AAS and other substance abuse include had encouraging results Adolescent Training and Learning to Avoid Steroids (ATLAS).

SUMMARY

Anabolic Steroid addiction is a problem worldwide, the effects of the condition are far reaching with medical and psychosocial negative consequences. Although Anabolic steroids do not induced the immediate gratification "high" as with the other drugs, Many users present with the classical addiction syndrome, Discontinuation of steroid use may reverse physical and psychological effects. However withdrawal leading to depression with suicidality is a serious effect and must be treated effectively. Comorbid substance use disorder also requires treatment.

ANABOLIC ANDROGENIC STEROIDS - PATIENT INFORMATION SHEET

What are Anabolic Steroids?

Anabolic steroids are artificial drugs that are similar but more potent than the male sex hormone testosterone. "Anabolic" means promotes muscle building, and "androgenic" refers to increases the male sexual and physical characteristics.

Do Anabolic Steroids have Legitimate Medical Uses?

yes. These drugs can be legally prescribed to treat conditions resulting from steroid hormone deficiency, such as delayed puberty, as well as debilitating diseases that result in loss of muscle mass, such as in cancer and AIDS . However due to their serious potential to cause harm they are considered controlled substances and in US are available by prescription only.

Are Anabolic Steroids Addictive?

Anabolic steroids don't cause "high" in the exact sense as with the use of other drugs. However they may lead to a classic picture seen in other addictions, where individuals use these drugs despite negative health consequences as well as negative effects on social and occupational or school functions. In addition these individuals spend large amount of time and resources in obtaining the drugs.

What are the Adverse Effects of Anabolic Steroids?

Anabolic steroids are like other pharmaceutical agents that are helpful when used for medical reasons under medical supervision. However they may leave to negative medical and emotional consequences if abused, like elevation blood pressure, increase in bad and decrease in good cholesterol, abnormal glucose level, abnormal liver function tests, baldness, benign and malignant tumors of liver, jaundice, abscesses at injection site, muscle hypertrophy, strokes in absence of risk factors, irritability, hostility, mania or depression, personality changes and psychosis. These medicines also affect directly the reproductive health leading to menstrual changes in females, increased breast sizes in men and sterility, low sperm count, reduced Testicle size. benign prostatic hypertrophy and masculine effects in women like voice changes. On occasions exchange of dirty needles has led to HIV/AIDS hepatitis B and C development.

What are the Withdrawal Effects Anabolic Steroids?

The withdrawal symptoms are generally seen in individuals who are heavy users, These include, anxiety, irritability, insomnia, decreased appetite or weight loss, sweating, headache, depression and in extreme cases suicidal thoughts and behaviors .

How is Anabolic Steroids Addiction is Treated?

There is no specific medicines that are known to treat that condition, Medicines are used to treat adverse medical and psychiatric consequences Counseling and education are valuable tools.

RESOURCES

http://www.dea.gov/druginfo/drug_data_sheets/Steroids.pdf

http://teens.drugabuse.gov/drug-facts/anabolic-steroids

CONFLICT OF INTEREST

The authors confirm that they have no conflict of interest to declare for this publication.

ACKNOWLEDGEMENTS

Declared none.

REFERENCES

[1] Kuhn CM. Anabolic steroids. Recent Prog Horm Res 2002; 57(1): 411-34. [http://dx.doi.org/10.1210/rp.57.1.411] [PMID: 12017555]

[2] Dawson RT. Drugs in sport - the role of the physician. J Endocrinol 2001; 170(1): 55-61. [http://dx.doi.org/10.1677/joe.0.1700055] [PMID: 11431137]

[3] Cohen J, Collins R, Darkes J, Gwartney D. A league of their own: demographics, motivations and patterns of use of 1,955 male adult non-medical anabolic steroid users in the United States. J Int Soc Sports Nutr 2007; 4: 12. [http://dx.doi.org/10.1186/1550-2783-4-12] [PMID: 17931410]

[4] Hall RC, Hall RC. Abuse of supraphysiologic doses of anabolic steroids. South Med J 2005; 98(5): 550-5. [http://dx.doi.org/10.1097/01.SMJ.0000157531.04472.B2] [PMID: 15954512]

[5] Kanayama Gen, *et al.* Anabolic-Androgenic Steroid Dependence: An Emerging Disorder. Addiction 2009; 104(12): 1966-78. [http://dx.doi.org/10.1111/j.1360-0443.2009.02734.x]

[6] Clement CL, Marlowe DB, Patapis NS, Festinger DS, Forman RF. Nonprescription steroids on the Internet. Subst Use Misuse 2012; 47(3): 329-41. [http://dx.doi.org/10.3109/10826084.2011.630225] [PMID: 22080724]

[7] Arvary D, Pope HG Jr. Anabolic-androgenic steroids as a gateway to opioid dependence. N Engl J Med 2000; 342(20): 1532. [http://dx.doi.org/10.1056/NEJM200005183422018] [PMID: 10819660]

[8] NIDA Research report Series , Anabolic Steroid abuse. Available from: https://www.drugabuse.gov/sites/default/files/rrsteroids_0.pdf , [accessed 04/12/2016];

[9] National Institute on Drug Abuse (NIDA). About anabolic steroid abuse. Nida Notes 2000; 15: 15.

[10] Brower KJ. Withdrawal from anabolic steroids. Curr Ther Endocrinol Metab 1997; 6: 338-43. [PMID: 9174765]

CHAPTER 9

Caffeine Related Use Disorder

Subhash C. Bhatia[1,*], **Venkata Kolli**[2], **Shashi K. Bhatia**[3] and **Usha Kanthety**[4]

[1] *Department of Psychiatry, Mental Health and Behavioral Sciences, Creighton University; Department VA Nebraska- Western Iowa Health Care System 4101 Woolworth Ave Omaha, NE 68105, USA*

[2] *Creighton- Nebraska Psychiatry Residency Training program, 3528 Dodge, Omaha, NE 68131, USA*

[3] *Departments of Psychiatry and Pediatrics, Division of Child and Adolescent Psychiatry, Creighton University, 3528 Dodge Omaha, NE 68131, USA*

[4] *Staff Physician, CHI, 1721, Colfax St, Schuyler, NE 68661, USA*

Abstract: 80% of the World's population consumes caffeine. Its impact on mental health often goes unrecognized. Caffeine use has comorbidity with other substance use disorders. Caffeine is a methylxanthine and exerts its actions by inhibiting adenosine receptors. Caffeine is a stimulant, mild to moderate use has beneficial effects like improving attention and concentration, but problem use can mimic anxiety, sleep and mood disorders. High dose caffeine can even result in death. In this chapter, we discuss common presentations of caffeine use disorders, their recognition and management. Caffeine withdrawal can present with mood disturbance and headaches, instant alleviation of these symptoms with caffeine perpetuates its use. Caffeine withdrawal with abrupt cessation typically lasts 2-4 days. Calculating baseline consumption and gradually reducing the caffeine intake can address the impact of the withdrawal symptoms.

Keywords: Adenosine, Caffeine, Caffeine intoxication, Caffeine use disorders, Caffeine withdrawal, Methylxanthine.

[*] **Corresponding author Subhash C. Bhatia:** Department of Psychiatry, Mental Health and Behavioral Sciences, Creighton University; Department VA Nebraska- Western Iowa Health Care System 4101 Woolworth Ave Omaha, NE 68105, USA; Tel: (402) 995-4315; Fax: (402)995-4240; Email: sub55@cox.net

KEY LEARNING POINTS

1. Caffeine is the most commonly used psychoactive substance around the globe. It exerts its stimulant action by inhibiting adenosine receptors.
2. Caffeine is consumed mainly as coffee. Also it is consumed in tea and caffeinated sodas. In adolescents energy drinks with high amounts of caffeine is a popular way to consume caffeine.
3. Caffeine related disorders are caffeine intoxication and caffeine withdrawal. Caffeine can cause anxiety like symptoms as well as caffeine induced sleep disorder.
4. Caffeine at low to moderate doses, *i.e.* less than 300mg, may cause positive effects like increased arousal and energy. However at high doses, *i.e.* greater than 400mg, it can cause negative effects like restlessness, nervousness and psychomotor agitation.
5. Caffeine can also cause cross sensitization with nicotine related disorders.

CLINICAL VIGNETTE

A 25-year-old male patient was referred by his employer for a psychiatric evaluation as he was observed to be "hyper". The patient reported that following departmental restructuring, he was taking on more responsibility. He reports experiencing poor sleep and anxiety about work. He reported being restless and exhibited pressured speech. He was sleeping only 4 hours and did not find sleep to be restful. He reported occasional panic attacks. He also reported seeing flashes of light occasionally. He has a history of smoking a pack of cigarettes a day but denied using illicit drugs. He reported drinking 5-6 cups of coffee and 2-3 energy drinks to promote alertness. He claimed that he tried to cut down on coffee. However on days he did not drink coffee he reported experiencing poor concentration, fatigue, headaches and depressed mood.

The patient reported recently he tried to cut down to 1-2 cups of coffee but had to increase his caffeine consumption to boost his energy to handle his increased work responsibilities and that it helped his fatigue and headaches also. He calculated his daily caffeine intake of 800-900 mg.

On physical examination, he had a pulse rate of 103. Urine toxicology screen was negative for illicit drugs. With this history and physical examination the patient was diagnosed to have caffeine related disorder.

Following education and advice on the role of coffee in his recent symptoms and work related problems, he reduced his caffeine intake by 25% every week. Following reduction of his coffee intake, he noted a gradual improvement in sleep, concentration and fatigue.

DISCUSSION OF THE VIGNETTE

Recognition

Caffeine is the most commonly used psychoactive substance in the world [1]. Because of its common use, most patients do not associate its effects with any psychiatric problems. Excess coffee consumption can present with insomnia, restlessness, anxiety and excitement such as that experienced by the patient in this vignette [1]. The patient has been using increasing amounts of caffeine to improve his attention and concentration and work performance. This resulted in the development of tolerance. Tolerance to insomnia took longer to develop.

DIAGNOSTIC CONSIDERATIONS

In this vignette our patient escalates his coffee consumption to cope with increased work related stress due to increased work responsibilities. This escalation also coincided with onset of his symptoms. Specifically, the patient was using caffeine to improve his concentration. Chronic use of caffeine leads to tolerance requiring higher amounts of caffeine to achieve the same results at work. Because of this he exhibited symptoms of caffeine intoxication manifesting as restlessness, rambling speech, excitement, insomnia and tachycardia [2]. Other common symptoms associated with caffeine intoxication are nervousness, flushed face, diuresis, gastrointestinal disturbances, muscle twitching, inexhaustibility and psychomotor agitation. When 5 or more of these symptoms are present and cause clinically significant distress or impairment a diagnosis of caffeine intoxication can be made [2].

This patient also experienced caffeine withdrawal characterized by symptoms such as poor concentration, fatigue and depressed mood, but noticed improvement of these symptoms with coffee consumption. Abrupt coffee cessation caused him headaches, fatigue, mood changes, and poor concentration. When 3 or more such symptoms are present causing marked impairment of social or occupational function, a diagnosis of caffeine withdrawal is made [2]. Even though the patient has been experiencing tolerance for the positive effects of caffeine, tolerance to insomnia developed later which is usually the case [3]. The symptoms of caffeine intoxication and withdrawal can mimic anxiety and/or mood disorders, but a careful history can delineate between the two. Caffeine induced anxiety disorder is sometimes difficult to distinguish from anxiety disorders. If anxiety worsens with caffeine consumption and improves with 1 week of caffeine abstinence, this points towards caffeine related anxiety disorder [3]. Caffeine related sleep disorder is diagnosed when sleep disturbance is a direct physiological consequence of caffeine consumption [2].

EPIDEMIOLOGY

80% of adults around the globe consume coffee [2]. In the United States average daily consumption of coffee per coffee drinker is about 280 mg [2 - 4]. Interestingly, caffeine users are nine times more likely to be cigarette smokers as well. Caffeine increases the metabolism of nicotine. In addition coffee drinkers have a higher prevalence of comorbid alcohol, benzodiazepine and other substance use disorders [5]. Caffeine increases body metabolism and sometimes is used by patients with eating disorders to lose weight [6]. Body builders use it to increase stamina and performance with exercise. In adolescents, the most common way of caffeine consumption is by drinking caffeinated soda. The second most common way is *via* energy drinks. Sleep is essential for brain development, it is not clear how sleep deprivation impacts adolescents [7].

CLINICAL PSYCHOPHARMACOLOGY

Caffeine inhibits adenosine receptors. There are 4 types of adenosine receptors *i.e.* A1, A2-a, A2-b and A3. The predominant stimulatory action is through blocking adenosine A1 and A2a receptors. Adenosine mediates the homeostatic sleep drive which is blocked by caffeine resulting in wakefulness as well as insomnia.

Caffeine reduces sleep efficiency and total sleep time. The highest concentration of A1 receptors is in hippocampus, cortex and cerebellum. A2A is hypothesized to potentiate dopamine neurotransmission and thereby through reward circuits may mediate addiction [8]. Adenosine A2A receptor gene (ADORA2A) is thought to cause variability in coffee consumption [9]. Caffeine also increases the turnover rate of various neurotransmitters, such as adrenergic action causing broncho-dilatation, increased blood pressure, increased gastric acid production and diuresis

Caffeine is metabolized by liver. Its half-life is 3-7 hours and is longer in those with hepatic impairment [8]. In small doses, *i.e.* 20-200 mg, caffeine results in increased scores on self-rated scale for alertness, wellbeing, energy and concentration [10]. Positive effects of caffeine are increased energy expenditure, improved sports performance and reduced perception of fatigue [11]. In part the beneficial effect of caffeine by regular caffeine users is alleviation of withdrawal symptoms due to overnight abstinence [8].

MEDICAL EFFECTS OF CAFFEINE

Caffeine is a methylxanthine with effect similar to theophylline, a bronchodilator [5]. It also has pro-convulsive effects and sometimes used to lower seizure threshold in ECT [12]. Caffeine is thought to promote bone loss and increase risk of cerebrovascular disease [13, 14]. Caffeine ingestion at higher doses can trigger cardiac arrhythmia and even death. Serum level of caffeine greater than 25 mg/L and above is considered dangerous. Lethal dose of caffeine is considered to be about 12 grams [15]. Overdose of caffeine is due to overdose of caffeinated diet pills and energy drinks. Most of these deaths are in the younger age group. It is not clear what preexisting cardiac conditions predispose this age group to such a fatal outcome [16]. This risk has been amplified with the rising popularity of caffeine containing alcoholic beverages [17]. Even though caffeine is used to treat headaches, rebound vasodilatation on withdrawal from caffeine can cause throbbing headaches [3, 18]. Caffeine has shown a promise in the treatment of Parkinson's disease. Its benefits are also being studied in other neurodegenerative disorders [19].

TREATMENT CONSIDERATIONS

Most symptoms of caffeine related disorders improve with abstinence and reduction. Caffeine withdrawal occurs in over 70% with abrupt cessation and 11% of this group notice significant impairment [2]. Caffeine withdrawal can occur if only 300mg of caffeine is consumed over 3 days; throbbing headache can occur 1-2 days following the last ingestion of caffeine. These withdrawal symptoms improve in 30-60 minutes following caffeine consumption [3]. Patients with anxiety and depression have a higher propensity to experience withdrawal headaches. Improvement of mood is seen in regular caffeine users when coffee is consumed in comparison to non-users. Withdrawl symptoms resolve in 2-4 days without active treatment. Some patients with insomnia may need a hypnotic for a short while.

Treatment of any caffeine related disorder should include education about its psychobiological effects. A weekly dairy of caffeine intake in mg equivalents helps the user understand their baseline consumption its progression or reduction. Manufacturers of caffeinated beverages may have the caffeine content listed on the label. If caffeine withdrawal symptoms on abrupt discontinuation are problematic, a reduction of daily consumption by 25% every week helps prevent a resurgence of withdrawal symptoms [3]. A coffee consumption goal should be made and follow-up visits are used to monitor progress. In individuals with repeated failures at attempts at reducing coffee consumption motivational enhancement therapy may be utilized.

CONCLUSION

Caffeine related disorders can mimic anxiety disorders more so in patients with preexisting psychiatric disorders. Careful history of caffeine consumption, psychoeducation, implementation of a caffeine reduction plan as well as monitoring progress may help alleviate the ill effects of caffeine use or its withdrawal.

PATIENT INFORMATION - EDUCATION SHEET

How Does Coffee Work?

Coffee's active ingredient is caffeine which works by inhibiting adenosine receptors. Adenosine is a neurochemical which builds up with fatigue. Caffeine helps alleviate fatigue by blocking adenosine's action on the receptors.

Does Coffee Cause Problems?

Caffeine does not cause problems when used in moderation. Consuming large quantities of coffee can make it difficult for you to fall asleep, can make you feel nervous, restless and make you have fast heart beat. Caffeine consumption in very large quantities has been associated with seizures, heart rhythm problems and even death.

Is Coffee Addictive?

Our body develops tolerance to caffeine when used regularly and experiences withdrawal effects when caffeine is stopped suddenly. It is sometimes abused by patients who want to loose weight. People addicted to caffeine might also be addicted to other substances like nicotine, alcohol and other illicit substances.

What Happens if I Suddenly Quit Drinking Coffee?

You can expect withdrawal effects like fatigue, throbbing headache and low mood. The degree and duration of withdrawal symptoms depends on your daily caffeine consumption. With moderate caffeine use withdrawal symptoms may last 2-4 days.

I Get Headaches when I don't Drink Coffee, What Should I Do?

Throbbing headache when you don't drink coffee is one of the withdrawal symptoms. It should improve in 2-4 days with abstinence.

I am Nervous. Is Caffeine the Cause?

Caffeine consumption can cause anxiety like symptoms or may exacerbate preexisting anxiety. If your anxiety improves significantly within a week of stopping caffeine intake your anxiety is very likely caffeine related.

I can't Cut Down Coffee, What Can I Do?

Cutting down caffeine consumption altogether at once can give you withdrawal symptoms. Look at product labels and calculate your daily caffeine intake for a week. Then try reducing by 25% every week.

I Use Several Energy Drinks to Improve Concentration. What is your Advice?

Caffeine enhances attention and concentration. However sleep disturbance associated with high caffeine consumption may result in poor concentration. This can be a vicious cycle.

Can Medication Help me to Quit Coffee Use?

There are no medications that can help you quit coffee use. It can be done gradually *i.e.* by decreasing your coffee intake 25% every week. If this does not work then working with your doctor or seeking help from a therapist might be beneficial.

CONFLICT OF INTEREST

The authors confirm that they have no conflict of interest to declare for this publication.

ACKNOWLEDGEMENTS

Declared none.

REFERENCES

[1] Winston AP, Hardwick E, Jaberi N. Neuropsychiatric effects of caffeine. Adv Psychiatr Treat 2005; 11(6): 432-9.
[http://dx.doi.org/10.1192/apt.11.6.432]

[2] American Psychiatric Association. Diagnostic and statistical manual of mental disorders. 5th ed., Arlington, VA: American Psychiatric Association 2013.

[3] Juliano LM, Griffiths RR. Caffeine-related disorders. Kaplan and Sadock's comprehensive textbook of psychiatry. 9th ed. USA: Lippincott Williams and Wilkins, Philadelphia 2009; pp. 1296-309.

[4] Lara DR. Caffeine, mental health, and psychiatric disorders. J Alzheimers Dis 2010; 20 (Suppl. 1): S239-48.
[PMID: 20164571]

[5] Reissig CJ, Strain EC, Griffiths RR. Caffeinated energy drinks--a growing problem. Drug Alcohol Depend 2009; 99(1-3): 1-10.
[http://dx.doi.org/10.1016/j.drugalcdep.2008.08.001] [PMID: 18809264]

[6] Baker JH, Mitchell KS, Neale MC, Kendler KS. Eating disorder symptomatology and substance use disorders: prevalence and shared risk in a population based twin sample. Int J Eat Disord 2010; 43(7): 648-58.
[http://dx.doi.org/10.1002/eat.20856] [PMID: 20734312]

[7] Temple JL. Caffeine use in children: what we know, what we have left to learn, and why we should worry. Neurosci Biobehav Rev 2009; 33(6): 793-806.
[http://dx.doi.org/10.1016/j.neubiorev.2009.01.001] [PMID: 19428492]

[8] Nehlig A. Are we dependent upon coffee and caffeine? A review on human and animal data. Neurosci Biobehav Rev 1999; 23(4): 563-76.
[http://dx.doi.org/10.1016/S0149-7634(98)00050-5] [PMID: 10073894]

[9] Cornelis MC, El-Sohemy A, Campos H. Genetic polymorphism of the adenosine A2A receptor is associated with habitual caffeine consumption. Am J Clin Nutr 2007; 86(1): 240-4.
[PMID: 17616786]

[10] Juliano LM, Griffiths RR. A critical review of caffeine withdrawal: empirical validation of symptoms and signs, incidence, severity, and associated features. Psychopharmacology (Berl) 2004; 176(1): 1-29.
[http://dx.doi.org/10.1007/s00213-004-2000-x] [PMID: 15448977]

[11] Astorino TA, White AC. Caffeine and Exercise Performance. In Preedy VR, Ed. Caffeine: Chemistry, Analysis. Function and Effects, RSC Publishers 2012; 2: 314.

[12] Coffey CE, Figiel GS, Weiner RD, Saunders WB. Caffeine augmentation of ECT. Am J Psychiatry 1990; 147(5): 579-85.
[http://dx.doi.org/10.1176/ajp.147.5.579] [PMID: 2183632]

[13] Hallström H, Byberg L, Glynn A, Lemming EW, Wolk A, Michaëlsson K. Long-term coffee consumption in relation to fracture risk and bone mineral density in women. Am J Epidemiol 2013; 178(6): 898-909.
[http://dx.doi.org/10.1093/aje/kwt062] [PMID: 23880351]

[14] Ding M, Bhupathiraju SN, Satija A, van Dam RM, Hu FB. Long-term coffee consumption and risk of cardiovascular disease: a systematic review and a dose-response meta-analysis of prospective cohort studies. Circulation 2013; 113 [Epub ahead of print].
[http://dx.doi.org/10.1161/CIRCULATIONAHA.113.005925] [PMID: 24201300]

[15] Jabbar SB, Hanly MG. Fatal caffeine overdose: a case report and review of literature. Am J Forensic Med Pathol 2013; 34(4): 321-4.
[http://dx.doi.org/10.1097/PAF.0000000000000058] [PMID: 24196726]

[16] Reissig CJ, Strain EC, Griffiths RR. Caffeinated energy drinks--a growing problem. Drug Alcohol Depend 2009; 99(1-3): 1-10.
[http://dx.doi.org/10.1016/j.drugalcdep.2008.08.001] [PMID: 18809264]

[17] Lau-Barraco C, Milletich RJ, Linden AN. Caffeinated alcohol consumption profiles and associations with use severity and outcome expectancies. Addict Behav 2014; 39(1): 308-15.

[18] Shapiro RE. Caffeine and headaches. Neurol Sci 2007; 28 (Suppl. 2): S179-83.
[http://dx.doi.org/10.1007/s10072-007-0773-5] [PMID: 17508167]

[19] Palacios N, Gao X, McCullough ML, *et al.* Caffeine and risk of Parkinson's disease in a large cohort of men and women. Mov Disord 2012; 27(10): 1276-82.
[http://dx.doi.org/10.1002/mds.25076] [PMID: 22927157]

Substance and Non Substance Related Addiction Disorders, 2017, 109-120

CHAPTER 10

Cannabis and Cannabinoid Use Disorders

Subhash C. Bhatia[1,*], **Shashi K. Bhatia**[2], **Venkata Kolli**[3] and **Jayakrishna Madabushi**[4]

[1] *Department of Psychiatry, Mental Health and Behavioral Sciences, Creighton University; Department VA Nebraska- Western Iowa Health Care System 4101 Woolworth Ave Omaha, NE 68105, USA*

[2] *Departments of Psychiatry and Pediatrics, Division of Child and Adolescent Psychiatry, Creighton University, 3528 Dodge Omaha, NE 68131, USA*

[3] *Creighton- Nebraska Psychiatry Residency Training Program, 3528 Dodge, Omaha, NE 68131, USA*

[4] *Baptist Health System, 517, Crowne Woods Drive, Birmingham, AL, 35244 USA*

Abstract: Cannabis or marijuana also called pot, grass, weed, herb *etc.* is derived from flowers, leaves, stem or seeds of cannabis sativa plant. It is consumed by smoking or mixing it with foods and beverages. Hashish is a resinous material made from cannabis plant . Cannabis and illicit synthetic THC compounds like "spice" K2" have similar psychoactive effects which are mediated through binding with cannabinoid receptor CB1. Whereas binding with CB2 receptors impacts immunity. Anandamides are the endogenous ligands for these receptors. THC is lipophilic and is deposited in fatty tissue and can be detected in the urine in chronic cannabis users for up to 30 days. THC synthetic compounds, Dronabinol (Marinol) and Nabilone (Cesamet) are approved for medicinal use in oncology, ophthalmology and AIDS. CB1 receptors binding in hippocampus causes short-term memory problems whereas binding in nucleus accumbens causes euphoria. Psychiatric disorders are mood and anxiety disorders. Psychosis is also reported. Genetic factors, as evidenced by twin studies, contribute from 30 to 80% variance to this risk. There are no pharmacological treatments approved for cannabis withdrawal. Short-term symptomatic treatment with non-benzodiazepine anxiolytics, antidepressants, or hypnotics may be considered. Cognitive-behavioral, motivational enhancement and family therapy, contingency management and self-help groups are valuable psychosocial treatment options.

* **Corresponding author Subhash C. Bhatia:** Department of Psychiatry, Mental Health and Behavioral Sciences, Creighton University; Department VA Nebraska- Western Iowa Health Care System 4101 Woolworth Ave Omaha, NE 68105, USA; Tel/Fax: (402)995-4315/(402)995-4240; Email: sub55@cox.net

Key words: Anadamides, Cannabinoid receptors CB1 and CB2, Cannabis, Grass, Hashish, Hemp, Herb, Herbal Incense, K2, Marijuana, Pot, Spice, Synthetic Cannabinoids, THC, Weed.

KEY LEARNING POINTS

1. The main psychoactive substance in cannabis is delta-9-tetrahydrocannabinol (THC). It exerts its psychoactive effect through cannabinoid receptor CB1.
2. Cannabis is consumed in a variety of ways; smoking has a faster onset, with three times more potency than oral use and is the most common route of consumption.
3. Cannabis related disorders are: cannabis use disorder, cannabis intoxication, cannabis withdrawal and cannabis-induced psychosis, anxiety, sleep disturbance and delirium.
4. Cannabis- induced disorders are more prevalent in patients suffering from other psychiatric disorders.
5. Treatment options include treatment of comorbid psychiatric disorders, motivational enhancement therapy, cognitive-behavioral therapy, contingency management and family based interventions.
6. Synthetic cannabinoid agonists have been available in Europe since 2004 and are now available in most other countries, under the street brand names K2 and Spice.

CLINICAL VIGNETTE

A 17-year-old male was brought to the clinic by his mother, following a recent history of poor academic performance. She feared that her son is depressed as he appeared more withdrawn, and had been sleeping and eating more. He had been missing school lately, and his grooming and hygiene had declined. On questioning, the patient admitted to yearlong difficulties with attention, concentration and memory. As a result, his grades have dropped from A's and B's to D's and F's. He denied any depression and reported feeling "great". His attention span and recall were impaired. He reported feeling anxious and had occasional panic attacks. He did not exhibit symptoms of psychosis. He denied any illicit drug use.

Physical examination was positive for conjunctival injection and a pulse rate of 103. Urine toxicological screen tested positive for carboxy-tetrahydrocannabinol. When the patient was confronted with the positive urine drug screen for cannabis, he admitted to smoking marijuana about 2 hours ago. He stated that he had been smoking about 6-8 "joints" daily for a year. He did not feel that cannabis use was a problem. He admitted to experiencing irritability, nervousness; sleep problems and restlessness when he did not smoke "pot". A motivation enhancement approach was used, discussing the consequences of use with benefits of change. Relaxation exercises and distraction techniques were utilized to cope with withdrawal. Random urine drug screen for THC was instituted with a reward of his favorite comic book contingent on negative urine drug screen. During one year follow up patient reported using marijuana once.

DISCUSSION OF THE VIGNETTE

Recognition

Cannabis (also called marijuana) is the most widely used illicit drug in the United States. Owing to its illicit status, patients are often not truthful about this drug use. THC is lipophilic, and deposits in the adipose tissue with chronic use and is slowly released. Hence cannabis can be detected with routine urine drug screening for up to 30 days following cessation of chronic use, and up to 3 days following acute use. Acute intoxication, as noted in our patient, may cause conjunctival injection, tachycardia, and increased appetite; whereas withdrawal symptoms include irritability, nervousness, sleep problems and restlessness. The psychoactive effects of THC are mediated through binding with cannabinoid receptor CB1. Binding to cannabinoid receptors in the hippocampus causes short-term memory difficulties. This negatively impacts cognitive functioning causing impairment of academic achievement. The statement of feeling "great" in our patient was likely to be related to binding of THC with cannabinoid receptors in nucleus accumbens, a reward center in the brain.

DIAGNOSTIC CONSIDERATIONS

Cannabis use disorder is diagnosed through history from the patient and collateral resources. Physical and mental status examination and urine drug screen aids in its recognition and diagnosis. Some patients minimize or deny its use, owing to its illegal status. In those circumstances, urine or saliva drug screen for THC is extremely valuable. Confirmation testing of positive THC screen is through gas chromatography or mass spectrometry. Hair and nail analysis for THC may be of value if there is long-term exposure to cannabis [1]. In DSM-5 [2] Cannabis related disorders, are sub classified as Cannabis use disorder, Cannabis Intoxication, Cannabis Withdrawal, Other cannabis use disorders (includes cannabis induced sleep, anxiety and psychotic disorders) and unspecified cannabis use disorders. Functional polymorphism of dopamine metabolizing enzyme catechol-o-methyl transferase is thought to mediate development of cannabis-induced psychosis [3]. CAGE questionnaire, an alcohol use disorders screening tool, can also be adapted for cannabis use disorders (c-cut down, ration or limit cannabis use; A-angered or annoyed easily when questioned about cannabis use; G-Guilt about its use and due to consequences of its use; E-eye opener, often smoking first "joint" upon awakening in the morning [4]. Severity of Dependence Scale (SDS) with five items and separate scoring norms for adolescents and adults is a reliable and valid screening instrument for cannabis use disorder [5].

EPIDEMIOLOGY

Cannabis or marijuana is described by different names such as pot, grass, weed, herb *etc.* and is derived from flowers, leaves, stem or seeds of cannabis sativa plant. Smoking with pipes, water pipes, hand-rolled cigarettes (joints) and mixture of tobacco and cannabis in cigars (blunts) are common methods of marijuana use. Other ways to consume cannabis is by mixing it with foods and beverages. Hashish is a resinous material made from cannabis plant and is used more commonly in Europe.

Cannabis is the most widely used illicit drug in the United States. The 2010 National Survey on Drug Use and Health (NSDUH) [6] stated that 17.4 million Americans used this drug in the past-month; of these, 76.8 percent were current users. In the adult population, cannabis use is common in males than females, but this gender difference is less prominent in adolescents. Cannabis is considered a 'gateway' drug and cannabis use before the age of 15 years is a significant predictor of future cannabis or other illicit substance use [2, 7]. Early cannabis use is often associated with co-occurring psychiatric disorders in young adults [2]. About 30% of adolescents using cannabis also experience comorbid anxiety, depression and posttraumatic stress disorder, and about 60% have conduct disorder and/or attention-deficit/hyperactivity disorder [2]. In 2011, the percentages of 8th, 10th and 12th graders using cannabis in the past and in the current year, respectively, were 12.5 and 7.2; 28.8 and 17.6 and 36.4 and 22.6 [8]. Cannabis use also contributed to increased emergency room visits. In both adolescent and adult Native and Alaskan Americans, the prevalence of cannabis is higher than any other ethnic groups in the US.

Psychiatric disorders associated with cannabis use disorder are major depressive disorder, anxiety disorder, bipolar I disorder, and posttraumatic stress disorder [9 - 11]. The presence of a preexisting psychiatric disorder increases the risk of cannabis use. The other risk factors for cannabis use are conduct disorder, socio-cultural and economic factors, easy availability of cannabis and family dysfunction. Genetic factors, as evidenced by twin studies, contribute from 30 to 80% variance to this risk [2].

CLINICAL PSYCHOPHARMACOLOGY

THC is the main psychoactive chemical in cannabis. When cannabis is smoked absorption *via* large surface area in the lungs, rapidly produces intoxication, characterized by euphoria, impaired motor coordination, impaired time sense, anxiety, impaired judgment and social withdrawal. In addition, there is the presence of conjunctival injection, increased appetite and dry mouth [2]. The onset of action is relatively slower if cannabis is ingested with food or beverages.

The human brain and body have an abundance of cannabinoid receptors (CB1 and CB2). CB1 is present in the neurons. The role of CB2 receptor in addiction is not clearly understood but is preponderant in the microglia and is thought to have an immunologic function [12]. Pain relieving properties are *via* cannabis action at

CB1, CB2 and VR1 receptors [13, 14]. Anandamides are endogenous cannabinoid ligands for these receptors [12]. Anandamides are akin to neurotransmitters and play an important role in normal brain development and function [15]. THC binding to CB1 and CB2 cannabinoid receptors disrupts their normal function and causes various symptoms of cannabis intoxication. Cannabis induced release of dopamine in the nucleus accumbens causes euphoria or "high", and binding in the cerebellum and basal ganglia leads to impaired coordination and impaired time sense [16]. Action at the brainstem causes an anti-nausea effect, and binding at amygdala explains anxiety, panic or fear symptoms [16]. Binding at hippocampal region cause cannabis related short-term memory problems and at hypothalamus explain increased appetite and sexual behavior [16]. Increased heart rate and conjunctival injection are part of acute intoxication. Ingestion of large quantities can cause delirium and psychosis. Long-term chronic cannabis use has a cumulative effect, leading to addiction, respiratory symptoms if smoked, mood, anxiety and psychotic symptoms. There are also reports of cannabis related apathy called amotivational syndrome. Positron Emission Tomography (PET) Fluorodeoxyglucose (FDG) imaging studies in chronic cannabis users showed lower cerebellar FDG metabolism in cannabis users than controls [17]. This may explain the lack of coordination and change in time sense since the cerebellum is linked to internal timing function.

Synthetic cannabinoid recreational use that started in Europe has now spread to many other countries. They are called K2 or Spice *etc* and have been sold as "Herbal Incense". These compounds mimic the effect of THC by binding to cannabinoid receptors. On 1 March 2011, five synthetic cannabinoids (JWH-018, JWH-073; CP-47,497, JWH-200 and cannabicyclohexanol) were placed on Schedule 1 of Controlled Substance Act, making their possession and use illegal in the United States. In July 2012, the Synthetic Drug Abuse Prevention Act of 2012 was signed in to law in the USA. Under this law, all synthetic cannabis products were placed under Schedule I. There has not been systematic research about the effects of these synthetic compounds. Case reports relating to abuse of these compounds causing psychosis have been reported [18].

Medical Marijuana has been legalized in 16 states and District of Columbia in the USA, because of scientific information that cannabis contains active substances with therapeutic benefit for mitigating pain, stimulating appetite, and reducing intraocular pressure in glaucoma. In the US, there are two FDA approved synthetic THC compounds, dronabinol (Marinol) and nabilone (Cesamet) for medicinal use for nausea in patients on chemotherapy and wasting syndrome due to Acquired Immune Deficiency Syndrome (AIDS). Recently a mouth spray (Sativex) that contains synthetic THC and cannabidiol has become available in the UK and Canada and is in the process of getting FDA approval in the United States for cancer related and neuropathic pain, and spasticity in multiple sclerosis.

MEDICAL EFFECTS WITH CANNABIS

Chronic smoking of marijuana puts patients at risk for chronic bronchitis, chronic obstructive pulmonary disease, emphysema and cancer [6], and has a negative effect on pulmonary function. Cannabis smoke contains 3.8 times more tar and 50% more carcinogenic hydrocarbons than tobacco [19]. Smoking both cannabis and tobacco exposes smoker to greater risk for cancer than either alone. There is some evidence that cannabis use may also negatively impacts the immune system. Cannabis is considered to be teratogenic and may result in a smaller size fetus and a low birth weight.

TREATMENT CONSIDERATIONS

The treatment settings for cannabis use disorders are very similar to treatment for other substance use disorders. Based on assessment dependent needs, treatment may be rendered in outpatient, residential or inpatient settings. Residential care may be appropriate for patients who, while not present danger to self or others, have a desire to quit and have failed outpatient treatment multiple times, have a limited social support system, or live in an environment that is not conducive to recovery. Inpatient treatment is warranted for patients who are a danger to self or others, or who have serious mental illness. Majority of patients can be treated as outpatients. Payee or a guardian might help ensure that their public assistance is not diverted towards illicit drugs. Population based public policy based on demand, supply and harm reduction with cannabis use is required.

PHARMACOLOGICAL INTERVENTIONS

There are no pharmacological treatments approved for cannabis withdrawal. Short-term symptomatic treatment with non-benzodiazepine anxiolytics, antidepressants, or hypnotics may be considered. Longer-term psychotropic medications may be considered if there is co-occurring psychiatric disorder. Effective treatment of co-occurring psychiatric disorders reduces cannabis use. Patients experiencing nicotine withdrawal treatment considerations for tobacco use disorder as described in chapter two may be considered. A randomized controlled study of gabapentin on cannabis use, withdrawal and executive function deficits has shown promise [20].

PSYCHOLOGICAL INTERVENTIONS

1. Cognitive behavioral therapy (CBT) in useful in the management of cannabis related disorders. Similar to other substance use disorders, patients with cannabis related disorders experience irrational thoughts and faulty drug use behaviors that CBT can help address. CBT helps with management of negative moods, reducing craving, development of strategies at reducing cannabis use and maintaining abstinence.
2. Motivational enhancement therapy (MET) uses principles of expressing empathy, developing discrepancy, rolling with resistance and supporting self-efficacy. Clinician uses skills to affirm, listen, reflect and summarize. Assessing for stage of change, *i.e.* pre contemplation, contemplation, preparation, action, maintenance and relapse, is useful in assessing as to where the patient is in the recovery process.
3. Contingency management (CM) is based on pairing cannabis abstinence evidenced by a negative urine drug screen, with a reward (cash, voucher or a product) is useful in reducing recidivism. They should be based on a contract and sustainable funding source.
4. Family therapy improves communication in the family and promotes positive outcomes.

SOCIAL INTERVENTIONS

Marijuana Anonymous (MA) and Narcotic Anonymous are similar to Alcoholic

Anonymous (AA). They are spirituality based 12 step programs. A peer support from a sponsor helps promote the recovery process.

SUMMARY

Cannabis and synthetic compounds mimicking THC effects pose a significant public health problem. Public policy addressing supply, demand and harm reduction is essential. Their use negatively impacts neuropsychological, social, occupational and physical health. Its use during formative years of children and adolescents is very problematic leading to use of other illicit drugs and long-term consequences. Availability of evidence based bio-psychosocial-spiritual treatment can reduce demand for its illicit use.

CANNABIS-RELATED DISORDERS- PATIENT EDUCATION SHEET

What is Cannabis?

Cannabis or marijuana is a greenish gray mixture of shredded dry leaves, stems, seeds and/or flowers of the Cannabis Sativa plant. The active mind altering ingredient in cannabis is delta-9-tetrahydrocanabinol or THC.

What is a Spice?

This is a synthetic product, which mimics the action of THC. This is also called K2 and is sold as “herbal incense”. In the US these products are Schedule I under the Controlled Substances Act, which makes it illegal to possess or use.

What are Symptoms of Cannabis Intoxication?

These include euphoria, motor in coordination with problems in operating machinery or motor vehicle, anxiety, sense of slow time, impaired judgment, anxiety, social withdrawal, rapid heartbeat, dry mouth, increase appetite, and even hallucinations.

What are the Withdrawal Effects of Cannabis Use?

The withdrawal symptoms are generally seen in individuals who are heavy users of cannabis. These include nervousness or anxiety, irritability, anger and aggression, insomnia, disturbing dreams, decreased appetite or weight loss, depression, shakes, tremors, sweating, fever, chills, headache and abdominal pain *etc*.

Is Cannabis Addictive?

Yes, it can be especially addictive if its use starts before age 15, if the person has a family history of cannabis related disorder or if the individual resorts to heavy use and has another mental disorder.

What Medical Complications can be Caused by Cannabis?

Cannabis when smoked can have similar short and long term complications, as with tobacco.

Can Cannabis Use Cause a Nervous Breakdown?

Yes. Cannabis intoxication can cause confusion. In addition cannabis can induce psychosis, which is more likely if there is a family history of psychosis.

Can Cannabis Use Disorder be Inherited?

Both genes and environment play a part. Genes contribute up to an 80% hereditable cannabis use risk.

How is Cannabis Related Disorder Diagnosed?

Clinicians obtain history from patient and collateral sources, conduct physical and mental status evaluation and utilize current diagnostic criteria. Detection and confirmation of THC in urine, saliva or in nails and hair strengthen the diagnostic probability.

How is Cannabis Use Disorders Treated?

There are no specific medications for cannabis use disorder treatment except in patients who also happen to have other mental illnesses. Individual, group and family therapy as well as 12-step AA programs with a sponsor are valuable options.

Are there Prescription based THC Products? What are their Benefits?

There are two FDA approved products under trade names Marinol and Cesamet, which can be prescribed for nausea in patients going through cancer chemotherapy and for wasting syndrome in AIDS victims.

CONFLICT OF INTEREST

The authors confirm that they have no conflict of interest to declare for this publication.

ACKNOWLEDGEMENTS

Declared none.

REFERENCES

[1] Bashford J. Screening and assessment of cannabis sue disorders. National Cannabis Prevention and Information Center (ncpic). Available from: http://ncpic.org.au/static/pdfs/background-papers/screening-and-assessment-for-cannabis-use-disorders.pdf 2013.

[2] Diagnostic and Statistical Manual of Mental Disorders. 5th ed., Arlington, VA: American Psychiatric Association 2013.

[3] Caspi A, Moffitt TE, Cannon M, *et al.* Moderation of the effect of adolescent-onset cannabis use on adult psychosis by a functional polymorphism in the catechol-O-methyltransferase gene: longitudinal evidence of a gene X environment interaction. Biol Psychiatry 2005; 57(10): 1117-27.

[4] Beck F, Legleye S. Measuring cannabis-related problems and dependence at the population level. In: Sznitman RS, Olsson B, Room R, Eds. A cannabis reader: global issues and local experiences; European Monitoring Centre for Drugs and Drug Addiction (EMCDDA) Monograph. 2008; Vol II.: pp. 36-7.

[5] Copeland J, Hall W. Choosing a diagnostic cut-off for cannabis dependence. Addiction 1998; 97: 1183-94.

[6] Office of Applied studies Results from 2010 National Survey on Drug Use and Health: Summary of National Findings HHS pub No (SMA) 11-4658. Rockville, MD: SAMHSA 2011.

[7] Fergusson DM, Boden JM, Horwood LJ. Cannabis use and other illicit drug use: testing the cannabis gateway hypothesis. Addiction 2006; 101(4): 556-69. [http://dx.doi.org/10.1111/j.1360-0443.2005.01322.x] [PMID: 16548935]

[8] Institute for Social Research. Monitoring the Future, 2011 (study Results). Ann Arbor, MI: University of Michigan 2012.

[9] Moore TH, Zammit S, Lingford-Hughes A, *et al.* Cannabis use and risk of psychotic or affective

mental health outcomes: a systematic review. Lancet 2007; 370(9584): 319-28.
[http://dx.doi.org/10.1016/S0140-6736(07)61162-3]

[10] Cougle JR, Bonn-Miller MO, Vujanovic AA, Zvolensky MJ, Hawkins KA. Posttraumatic stress disorder and cannabis use in a nationally representative sample. Psychol Addict Behav 2011; 25(3): 554-8.
[http://dx.doi.org/10.1037/a0023076] [PMID: 21480682]

[11] Arias F, Szerman N, Vega P, *et al.* Abuse or dependence on cannabis and other psychiatric disorders. Madrid study on dual pathology prevalence. Actas Esp Psiquiatr 2013; 41(2): 122-9.
[PMID: 23592072]

[12] Elkashef A, Vocci F, Huestis M, *et al.* Marijuana neurobiology and treatment. Subst Abus 2008; 29(3): 17-29.
[http://dx.doi.org/10.1080/08897070802218166] [PMID: 19042204]

[13] Jancsó G, Dux M, Oszlács O, Sántha P. Activation of the transient receptor potential vanilloid-1 (TRPV1) channel opens the gate for pain relief. Br J Pharmacol 2008; 155(8): 1139-41.
[http://dx.doi.org/10.1038/bjp.2008.375] [PMID: 18997813]

[14] Starowicz K, Malek N, Przewlocka B. Cannabinoid receptors and pain. WIREs Member Transp Signal 2013; 2: 121-32.
[http://dx.doi.org/10.1002/wmts.83]

[15] Battista N, Di Tommaso M, Bari M, Maccarrone M. The endocannabinoid system: an overview. Front Behav Neurosci 2012; 6: 9.
[http://dx.doi.org/10.3389/fnbeh.2012.00009] [PMID: 22457644]

[16] US Department of Health and Human Services, National Institutes of Health, National Institute on Drug Abuse. 2012.

[17] 17.Volkow ND, Gillespie H, Mullani N, Tancredi L, Grant C, Valentine A, and Hollister L. Brain Glucose Metabolism in Chronic Marijuana Users During Baseline and During Marijuana Intoxication. Psychiatry Res 1996; 67: 29-38.
[http://dx.doi.org/10.1016/0925-4927(96)02817-X] [PMID: 8797240]

[18] Hurst D, Loeffler G, McLay R. Psychosis associated with synthetic cannabinoid agonists: a case series. Am J Psychiatry 2011; 168(10): 1119-9.
[http://dx.doi.org/10.1176/appi.ajp.2011.11010176] [PMID: 21969050]

[19] Wu TC, Tashkin DP, Djahed B, Rose JE. Pulmonary hazards of smoking marijuana as compared with tobacco. N Engl J Med 1988; 318(6): 347-51.
[http://dx.doi.org/10.1056/NEJM198802113180603] [PMID: 3340105]

[20] Mason BJ, Crean R, Goodell V, *et al.* A Proof-of-Concept Randomized Controlled Study of Gabapentin: Effects on Cannabis Use, Withdrawal and Executive Function Deficits in Cannabis-Dependent Adults. Neuropsychopharmacology advance on line publication,29 February 2012; doi:10.1038/npp.2012.14

CHAPTER 11

Ecstasy Substance Use Disorder

Subhash C. Bhatia[1,*] and **Aly Hassan**[2]

[1] *Department of Psychiatry, Mental Health and Behavioral Sciences, Creighton University; Department VA Nebraska- Western Iowa Health Care System 4101 Woolworth Ave Omaha, NE 68105, USA*

[2] *Phoenix VA Health Care System, Department of Psychiatry, University of Arizona, Phoenix College of Medicine, Gilbert VA Clinic, 3285 S Val Vista Drive, Gilbert AZ 85925, USA*

Abstract: Ecstasy or 3, 4- methylenedioxymethamphetamine also called a club drug because of its use in "rave" parties has both stimulant and psychedelic effects. Stimulant effect which precedes psychedelic effect causes euphoria. In addition through release of oxytocin prosocial and empathic behavior as well as sense of intimacy is experienced. The psychedelic effect causes distortion of sensory perceptions. This drug is popular with adolescents and young adults and often associated with prolonged weekend "rave" parties. Its use causes depletion of serotonin which may cause depression and suicidal behavior. Depression may also be caused by "crash" from stimulant effect. With intoxication of ecstasy patient often experiences autonomic effects like elevated blood pressure, elevated temperature, cardiac arrhythmia, and panic attacks. In addition patient may experience headaches, vertigo, seizure and loss of consciousness. For intoxication treatment is supportive and symptomatic. There are no specific medications for its treatment. Psychosocial interventions like cognitive behavioral therapy, social and coping skills training and treatment of comorbid psychiatric disorder are very valuable options.

Keywords: Club drug, Ecstasy, MDMA, Oxytocin release, Pro social and pro empathy drug, Rave parties.

* **Corresponding author Subhash C. Bhatia:** Department of Psychiatry, Mental Health and Behavioral Sciences, Creighton University; Department VA Nebraska- Western Iowa Health Care System 4101 Woolworth Ave Omaha, NE 68105, USA; Tel/Fax: (402) 995-4315/(402) 995-4240; E-mail: sub55@cox.net

Subhash C. Bhatia (Ed.)

KEY POINTS

1. Ecstasy or MDMA is an acronym for (3, 4-methylenedioxymethamphetamine) is so called "club drug". It has both stimulant and psychedelic properties. The former effect gives euphoria, interpersonal warmth and sense of intimacy and the later relates to distortion of sensory perceptions and time. It is also reported to provide enhanced pleasure through tactile experiences.
2. MDMA synthesized in 1900s in Germany. In 1970s some psychiatrists used MDMA as a psychotherapy tool without evidence of its benefits.
3. MDMA is considered empathomimetic due to its indirect activation of serotonin system and increased release of oxytocin.
4. In 1985 because of no medical benefits but significant abuse potential MDMA it was classified as schedule I drug. MDMA is an addictive drug and tolerance can happen too.
5. MDMA use became popular with adolescents and young adults in "rave", all night weekend nightclub parties. However its use has spread to other settings and demographics.
6. MDMA is neurotoxic to serotonin neurons and therefore can deplete serotonin leading to depression usually during early part of week when the effect of drug has worn off and person crashes which may increase suicidality so called "Tuesday Suicide".
7. Undesirable effects like anxiety, irritability, restlessness, sadness, impulsivity, aggression, sleep problems, reduced appetite and interest in sex and reduction in mental ability may last for up to o one week.
8. Intoxication and overdose with MDMA may cause elevated blood pressure, dizziness and fainting episodes, panic attacks, loss of consciousness and seizures.

CLINICAL VIGNETTE

A group of men brought a young man who appeared restless with heavy breathing to the local hospital ER in the early morning hours. A friend volunteered to report that they were in a rave party that lasted nine hours. He reported that his friend until half an hour ago seemed fine but started to complain of headache and became slow and sluggish and his speech became slow, also. The young man reported that at this site of the party "they were selling the bottle of water for 6 dollars" and water from outside was not allowed. Therefore his consumption of fluids was limited. He added that his friend may have used Ecstasy and marijuana which he occasionally does. He was not sure however about the amount of Ecstasy the patient consumed. The vital signs were as follows: temperature 103, pulse rate 140, BP 148/92 and respiration rate 29, dry skin and tongue was suggestive of dehydration which was later confirmed by urine specific gravity. Patient was given IV saline to hydrate him. Gastric lavage with activated charcoal was done. Liver functions were normal. For sedation diazepam 5 mg was given orally.

DISCUSSION OF THE VIGNETTE

Based on history and urine drug screen Ecstasy use disorder was diagnosed. Gastric lavage with activated charcoal was performed. Elevated temperature was a symptom of Ecstasy use and dehydration. If untreated, this may progress to hyperthermia. Sodium level was normal. Agitation is treated with a benzodiazepine in this case diazepam which benefited agitation. Low potency neuroleptics like chlorpromazine should be avoided due to its intrinsic anticholinergic effects which can further elevate temperature. Due to the hepatotoxicity of MDMA hepatic functions should be evaluated which were normal in this patient. Blood pressure and elevated heart rate due to noradrenergic effects should be monitored.

NEUROPSYCHOPHARMACOLOGY

MDMA releases monoamine neurotransmitters (serotonin, norepinephrine and dopamine) in the brain [1] causes indirect activation of serotonergic system. Through 5HT 1A receptors MDMA increases release of oxytocin which promotes prosocial behavior [2, 3]. Oxytocin is typically released during hugging, sexual orgasm as well as child birth. Long term use of MDMA can cause neurotoxic effects on serotonin neurons causing depletion [4, 5] leading to depression and suicidal behavior. This is more often during mid-week [6]. Therapeutic effects of MDMA in Anxiety disorders are hypothesized to be due to increased oxytocin, increase in ventromedial prefrontal activity and as a result decrease in amygdala activity as well as increased norepinephrine release and cortisol which facilitates emotional engagement in avoidant individuals [7].

MDMA INTOXICATION

Psychological Effects

MDMA reaches peak concentrations in 1.5 and 3 hours [8] after ingestion, faster after smoking. The effects may last from 3-5 hours. Serum level decreases to half of its peak level in approximately 8 hours [9].

Stimulant effects of MDMA are preceded by psychedelic effect. This leads to euphoria, increased willingness to communicate, increased energy, feelings of comfort, sense of belonging and closeness to others, feelings of love and empathy, increased awareness of music, enhanced sensory perception and enjoyment of tactile experiences, anxiety, difficulty concentrating and impulsive aggressive behavior. During the crash depression and suicidality may manifest.

Physical Effects

Jaw clenching (trismus), tongue and cheek chewing, and teeth grinding, muscle tension and cramping, sweating, increase in body temperature, increased blood pressure, cardiac arrhythmias, hyperthermia, dehydration, hyponatremia, nausea and vomiting, headaches, dizziness, loss of balance, vertigo, seizures and loss of consciousness.

EPIDEMIOLOGY

At least once in a life time use of MDMA among individuals aged 12 years or older was 10.2 million in 2000, 11 million in 2004 and 14.2 million in 2009. Also in 2004, 450,000 individuals in this age group used it during the past month. Although the drug started as popular among young white urbanites, its use spread to a broader range of ethnic groups and among populations outside the rave club scene [10].

DIAGNOSTIC CONSIDERATIONS

In DSM-5 [11] Ecstasy use disorder is described under Other Hallucinogen Use Disorders; Other Hallucinogen Intoxication; Hallucinogen Persisting Perception Disorder; Other Hallucinogen-Induced Disorders and Unspecified Hallucinogen-Related Disorder.

The diagnosis of MDMA intoxication is made by history of drug intake and/or analysis of unused drug. Most signs and symptoms are not specific to MDMA, but resemble those of stimulants and hallucinogens. MDMA has been recently included in the department of transportation urine drug screen basic panel. MDMA may have withdrawal symptoms that resemble a mild form of stimulant withdrawal or "crash", with depression, anxiety, fatigue, and difficulty concentrating. There is also risk of suicide during withdrawal.

TREATMENT

Pharmacotherapy

There are no specific pharmacological treatments for MDMA abuse or addiction. In some patients, treatment of autonomic symptoms, hyperthermia, anxiety or depression is warranted.

Psychosocial Interventions

During intoxication and withdrawal, patient's safety with the help of friends or family should be assured. A suicidal patient may require hospitalization.

Cognitive behavioral therapy designed to modify a patients thinking, as well as, social skills training and coping skills training can be helpful.

MDMA - PATIENT EDUCATION SHEET

What is Ecstasy?

The acronym for this chemical is MDMA. In drug of abuse culture it is also called an E, X or XTC. It is an illegal club drug consumed in 'rave' parties usually by adolescents and young adults.

How Does it Work?

It has effects both of amphetamine and hallucinogen. The amphetamine effect gives a good feeling whereas the psychedelic effect causes hallucinations, distortions of perceptions and time sense like it is with LSD.

What are the Effects of this Drug?

It cause both physical symptoms like fast heartbeat, loss of appetite, chills, sweating, fever, high blood pressure as well as psychological symptoms of anxiety, irritability, angry out bursts and depression.

Is this Drug Addictive?

Close to 50% of individuals develop dependence on the drug and crave to use it again. 60% of users report withdrawal symptoms like fatigue, depression and trouble concentrating.

How is the Addiction Treated?

There are no specific medications. Cognitive behavior therapy, coping and social skills training have benefit

Where I can Get More Information?

National Institute of drug Abuse (NIDA) web site:

www.drugabuse.gov

CONFLICT OF INTEREST

The authors confirm that they have no conflict of interest to declare for this publication.

ACKNOWLEDGEMENTS

Declared none.

REFERENCES

[1] Fitzgerald JL, Reid JJ. Effects of methylenedioxymethamphetamine on the release of monoamines from rat brain slices. Eur J Pharmacol 1990; 191(2): 217-20. [http://dx.doi.org/10.1016/0014-2999(90)94150-V] [PMID: 1982265]

[2] Dumont GJ, Sweep FC, van der Steen R, *et al.* Increased oxytocin concentrations and prosocial feelings in humans after ecstasy (3,4-methylenedioxymethamphetamine) administration. Soc Neurosci 2009; 4(4): 359-66. [http://dx.doi.org/10.1080/17470910802649470] [PMID: 19562632]

[3] Theodoridou A, Rowe AC, Penton-Voak IS, Rogers PJ. Oxytocin and social perception: oxytocin increases perceived facial trustworthiness and attractiveness. Horm Behav 2009; 56(1): 128-32. [http://dx.doi.org/10.1016/j.yhbeh.2009.03.019] [PMID: 19344725]

[4] Colado MI, O'Shea E, Granados R, Misra A, Murray TK, Green AR. A study of the neurotoxic effect of MDMA ('ecstasy') on 5-HT neurones in the brains of mothers and neonates following administration of the drug during pregnancy. Br J Pharmacol 1997; 121(4): 827-33. [http://dx.doi.org/10.1038/sj.bjp.0701201] [PMID: 9208155]

[5] Kish SJ, Furukawa Y, Ang L, Vorce SP, Kalasinsky KS. Striatal serotonin is depleted in brain of a human MDMA (Ecstasy) user. Neurology 2000; 55(2): 294-6. [http://dx.doi.org/10.1212/WNL.55.2.294] [PMID: 10908909]

[6] Curran HV, Travill RA. Mood and cognitive effects of +/-3,4-methylenedioxymethamphetamine (MDMA, 'ecstasy'): week-end 'high' followed by mid-week low. Addiction 1997; 92(7): 821-31. [PMID: 9293041]

[7] Johansen PO, Krebs TS. How could MDMA (ecstasy) help anxiety disorders? A neurobiological rationale. J Psychopharmacol (Oxford) 2009; 23(4): 389-91. [http://dx.doi.org/10.1177/0269881109102787] [PMID: 19273493]

[8] de la Torre R, Farré M, Ortuño J, *et al.* Non-linear pharmacokinetics of MDMA ('ecstasy') in humans. Br J Clin Pharmacol 2000; 49(2): 104-9. [http://dx.doi.org/10.1046/j.1365-2125.2000.00121.x] [PMID: 10671903]

[9] Farré M, Roset PN, Lopez CH, *et al.* Pharmacology of MDMA in humans. Ann N Y Acad Sci 2000; 914: 225-37. [http://dx.doi.org/10.1111/j.1749-6632.2000.tb05199.x] [PMID: 11085324]

[10] NIDA Research Report Series. National institute of drug Abuse 2006. NIH Publication Number 06-4728.

[11] American Psychiatric Association: Diagnostic and Statistical Manual of Mental Disorders, Fifth Edition. Arlington VA: American Psychiatric Association 2013.

CHAPTER 12

Hallucinogen-LSD Use Disorder

Subhash C. Bhatia[1,*] and **Aly Hassan**[2]

[1] *Department of Psychiatry, Mental Health and Behavioral Sciences, Creighton University; Department VA Nebraska- Western Iowa Health Care System 4101 Woolworth Ave Omaha, NE 68105, USA*

[2] *Phoenix VA Health Care System, Department of Psychiatry, University of Arizona, Phoenix College of Medicine, Gilbert VA Clinic, 3285 S Val Vista Drive, Gilbert AZ 85925, USA*

Abstract: LSD is the most potent hallucinogen. This as well as other hallucinogens have been used for religious rituals by Native Americans for centuries. LSD chemical structure has similarity to serotonin and works through post synaptic 5-HT2A receptor agonistic effects. LSD was first synthesized in late nineteen thirties. LSD intoxication significantly increases central autonomic activity leading to panic states, tachycardia, increased blood pressure and body temperature, pupillary dilatation, piloerection, tremor and hyperreflexia. The panic states, perceptual disturbances and flashbacks are often referred to as "trips". Patient may experience these "trips" long after cessation of its use. Subjective effects of LSD start with somatic symptoms followed by perceptual disturbances, lability of mood, depersonalization, altered sense of time, visual distortions, mixing of sensations like "seeing" smells and "hearing" colors. This mixing of sensations is called synesthesia. LSD is not addictive but tolerance to behavioral effects and cross tolerance to other hallucinogens drugs are reported. Acute intoxication results in somatic, perceptual and psychic effects. Some patients also relive these experiences through flashbacks even long after cessation of its use. No withdrawal symptoms are reported. Long -Term effects of LSD use may include psychosis, depression, paranoid delusions and flashbacks. The treatment therefore will consist of targeting the specific clinical syndrome like with SSRIs for depression, antipsychotics like chlorpromazine for psychosis and bad "trips". As with acute effects safety of the user must be assured and may require inpatient admission. Comorbid mental disorder should be treated to improve outcome. Cognitive behavioral therapy, social skills enhancement training can help to improve adaptive functions.

* **Corresponding author Subhash C. Bhatia:** Department of Psychiatry, Mental Health and Behavioral Sciences, Creighton University; Department VA Nebraska- Western Iowa Health Care System 4101 Woolworth Ave Omaha, NE 68105, USA; Tel/Fax: (402) 995-4315/(402) 995-4240; E-mail: sub55@cox.net

Keywords: DMT, Ergot derivative, Hallucinogen, LSD, LSD Trip, Lysergic Acid, MDA, Synesthesia.

KEY LEARNING POINTS

1. Hallucinogens include indole derivatives with structural similarities to serotonin. These are lysergic acid diethylamide (LSD), psilocybin, dimethyltryptamine (DMT). Other hallucinogens are substituted phenethylamines derivatives like mescaline, dimethoxymethylamphetamine (DOM), methylenedioxyamphetamine (MDA) and methyenedoxymethamphetamine (MDMA or Ecstasy). Phencyclidine (PCP) and cannabis. This chapter will primarily focus on LSD. PCP and cannabis are covered in other chapters.
2. LSD was first manufactured in 1938 from lysergic acid an ergot a fungus that grows on rye grain. In the USA its use became prevalent in the 1960's.
3. LSD is one of the most potent hallucinogens. Even 20 micrograms of the drug may manifest full behavioral effects; street doses range between 10-300 micrograms. Because of its high potency LSD it is applied to blotting paper and sold as pieces of it or applied to the back of postage stamps.
4. LSD is rapidly absorbed from the gastrointestinal track, easily crosses the blood brain barrier with behavioral effects manifesting within 60 minutes and peaking in 2-4 hours. The effects may last up to 12 hours.
5. The hallucinogenic activity of LSD and other serotonin class hallucinogens is possibly due to postsynaptic 5HT2A receptor agonism.
6. LSD significantly increases central autonomic activity. As a result the person may experience panic states, tachycardia, increased blood pressure and body temperature, pupillary dilatation, piloerection, tremor and hyperreflexia. The panic states, perceptual disturbances and flashbacks are often referred to as "trips". LSD is classified as Schedule I substance.
7. Subjective effects of LSD start with somatic symptoms followed by perceptual disturbances, changes in mood with lability, depersonalization, altered sense of time, visual distortions, mixing of sensations like "seeing" smells and "hearing" colors. This mixing of sensations is called synesthesia.

8. LSD is not considered an addictive drug. It lacks compulsive drug-seeking behavior.
9. With chronic use tolerance develops to behavioral effects but not to autonomic effects. Cross tolerance develops to mescaline and psilocybin but not to other drugs like PCP and cannabis.
10. There are no withdrawal symptoms following abrupt cessation of chronic use of LSD.

CLINICAL VIGNETTE

A twenty-one year old single white male presented to the office after discharge from the hospital. He stated that he has been having memory lapses. Prior to hospitalization he was found sitting on a residential patio. When residents of that house returned the person did not leave and therefore they called the police. He was arrested and ticked for trespassing. The police took him to the hospital rather than to the jail. When he woke up later that night in the hospital he stated he has no memory of that day. He had a similar experience about three months ago and doesn't recall what happened then either. On further questioning, he said he got into trouble at work last month because he missed a day of work and didn't realize it. He just got up one morning and went to work and was told he missed the day before and he couldn't remember the day before. It was just like it never happened. He is otherwise in good health. His Mini Mental Status Examination (MMSE) score today was 30/30. He was neurologically intact. Physical examination was normal. He worked as an electronics and computer sales person. He appears to be of average to above average intelligence. He denied the use of alcohol. He stopped using marijuana as his job performs random urine drugs screen. He stated he uses LSD frequently which he enjoys, it makes him hallucinate and provides him deeper insight about his own self. He first used LSD about four years ago. Since then he has used it every week or two. He denied craving about its use or spending lot of time in acquiring or using the drug. He stated that he has experienced LSD "trips" of variable intensity. He did not know the reason for variability in intensity or duration of "trips". He states he is a little "fuzzy" each time he comes "down" and that may be part of his memory problems. He denied illicit use of other drugs.

DISCUSSION OF CASE VIGNETTE

The patient was seen after the acute effects of LSD subsided. He presented with the subjective complaint of memory problems with no objective evidence of cognitive deficit. Our patient did not report craving.

EPIDEMIOLOGY

In 2007 in the USA over 22.7 million individuals twelve or older reported using LSD at least once during their lifetime. At that time the numbers for use in the last 12 months were fewer than 620,00. There was no change between 2006 and 2007 in the number initiating use of LSD in the past-year. DSM-5 [4] has listed diagnostic criteria for hallucinogen related disorders as: hallucinogen use disorder, hallucinogen intoxication, hallucinogen persisting perception disorder, other hallucinogen-induced disorders and unspecified hallucinogen-related disorder. In general the 12 month prevalence rate for hallucinogen use is reported to be higher among Native Americans and Alaska Natives compared to Caucasians, African Americans and Hispanics.

NEUROBIOLOGY OF LSD USE DISORDER

The exact mechanism of action of LSD and other hallucinogens is not known. LSD alters serotonergic transmission [1, 2] specifically through agonism of 5HT 2A receptors [3].

DIAGNOSTIC CONSIDERATIONS

DSM-5 has 10 diagnostic criteria for hallucinogen use disorder with Specifiers for early and sustained remissions or remission due to controlled environment. Severity is specified as mild, moderate and severe if number of symptoms present is respectively is 2-3, 4-5 or more than 6 [4].

LSD INTOXICATION SYNDROME

The acute effects of LSD are divided in to somatic, perceptual and psychological. Somatic symptoms occur first and are dizziness, paresthesias, weakness, tremor, and rapid heartbeat. Perceptual disturbances are alterations of visual and hearing senses. Psychological symptoms are rapid changes in emotions, anxiety, depression, visual illusion, visual distortions and visual hallucinations, alteration in sense of time and self, depersonalization, derealization, mixing of different senses, giving the user the feeling of hearing colors and seeing sounds is called synesthesia. Some LSD users experience intense terrifying thoughts of hopelessness, fear of losing control, fear of insanity and even death. LSD users often experience flashbacks related to reliving certain symptoms of LSD use up to a year later. These may occur suddenly and often without warning. Hallucinogen-induced persisting perceptual disorder (HPPD). This condition is diagnosed when the flashbacks are experienced episodically or continuously, it causes significant distress with impairment of social and occupational functioning. Most LSD users try to voluntarily decrease or stop its use. As stated earlier LSD is not an addictive drug and has no compulsive drug seeking behavior. However, LSD use may produce tolerance to its behavioral effects. As a result some users take larger quantity of the drug to replicate past intoxication related experiences. The dose dependent effects of LSD are mostly autonomic in nature like dilated pupils; raised body temperature and increased heart rate and blood pressure, profuse sweating, loss of appetite, drowsiness, dry mouth and tremors. There is no report of LSD associated withdrawal syndrome.

TREATMENT OF LSD USE AND LSD-INDUCED DISORDERS

Pharmacotherapy

There is no FDA approved treatment for acute effects of LSD use disorder. It requires prevention of physical harm to self or others, management of anxiety through reassurance, support and/or diazepam. Chlorpromazine is effective for LSD psychosis and the LSD "trip". Chlorpromazine can cause seizures by further lowering the seizure threshold specifically in patients using drugs contaminated with other substances also known to lower this threshold.

Long-term effects of LSD use may include psychosis, depression, paranoid delusions and flashbacks. The treatment therefore will consist of targeting the specific clinical presentation like SSRIs for depression, antipsychotics like chlorpromazine for psychosis and bad "trips". As with acute effects safety of the user must be assured. Comorbid mental disorder should be treated to improve outcome.

Psychosocial Interventions

Cognitive behavioral therapy, social skills training, social skills enhancement can help to improve adaptive functions.

SUMMARY

LSD and other hallucinogens have been used for religious rituals for centuries. Its chemical structure has similarity to serotonin and works through 5-HT2A receptor agonistic effects. This drug is generally not addictive but tolerance to behavioral effects and cross tolerance to other hallucinogen is known. Acute intoxication results in somatic, perceptual and psychic effects. Some patients also relive these experiences through flashbacks even long after cessation of its use. No withdrawal symptoms are reported.

LSD - PATIENT EDUCATION SHEET

What is LSD?

LSD is an ergot from a fungus which grows in grain like rye. LSD is a member of the hallucinogen class of street drugs. Its street name is acid. It is a very potent drug. Amounts as little as 10 micrograms may cause an acid trip. It was first discovered in 1938 and its street use started in the 1960s.

What Effects Does Acid Have?

The user experiences physical symptoms like a fast heartbeat, high blood pressure, large pupils, and tremor; psychological effects like scary feelings of dying, panic, seeing things which are not there, seeing distortions of time sense and things in the environment. Mixing of sensations like “seeing” sounds and smells and “hearing” colors.

What is an Acid Trip?

The user may relive effects of LSD weeks, months or years after quitting its use.

The effects are similar to when person used it for the first time and became intoxicated with it.

How Does LSD Cause these Effects?

LSD possibly works through a neurochemical in the brain called serotonin.

Is LSD Addictive?

It is not addictive since it does not associated with compulsive drug-seeking behavior. However it can cause tolerance and the user may take higher and higher amounts to achieve intoxication which can be extremely dangerous.

How is LSD Use Treated?

Patient who is intoxicated should be assessed for safety because this state may result in danger to self or others. Reassurance, minor and major tranquilizers may assist in mitigating symptoms of acute intoxication. Long-term treatment is similar to other substance use disorder *i.e.* individual or group counseling.

Where can I Get More Information?

You may access more information at:

http://www.drugabuse.gov/publications/drugfacts/hallucinogens-lsd-peyote-psilocybin-pcp

CONFLICT OF INTEREST

The authors confirm that they have no conflict of interest to declare for this publication.

ACKNOWLEDGEMENTS

Declared none.

REFERENCES

[1] Jacobs BL. How hallucinogenic drugs work. Am Sci 1987; 75: 386-92.

[2] Fantegrossi WE, Murnane KS, Reissig CJ. The behavioral pharmacology of hallucinogens. Biochem

Pharmacol 2008; 75(1): 17-33.
[http://dx.doi.org/10.1016/j.bcp.2007.07.018] [PMID: 17977517]

[3] Stahl SM. Stahl's essential psychopharmacology: neuroscientific basis and practical applications. 4th ed., New York: Cambridge University Press 2013.

[4] Diagnostic and Statistical Manual of Mental Disorders. 5th ed., Arlington, VA: American Psychiatric Association 2013.

CHAPTER 13

Inhalant Use Disorders

Aly Hassan[1], **Subhash C. Bhatia**[2,*] and **Shashi K. Bhatia**[3]

[1] *Phoenix VA Health Care System, Department of Psychiatry, University of Arizona, Phoenix College of Medicine, Gilbert VA Clinic, 3285 S Val Vista Drive, Gilbert AZ 85925, USA*

[2] *Department of Psychiatry, Mental Health and Behavioral Sciences, Creighton University; Department VA Nebraska- Western Iowa Health Care System 4101 Woolworth Ave Omaha, NE 68105, USA*

[3] *Departments of Psychiatry and Pediatrics, Division of Child and Adolescent Psychiatry, Creighton University, 3528 Dodge Omaha, NE 68131, USA*

Abstract: Inhalation of volatile hydrocarbon-based substances produces intoxication and pleasurable effects. Use of inhalants usually starts in adolescence ages 12 to 17 often precedes use of tobacco, alcohol and illicit substances. It decreases gradually after the age of 20 years. These substances are lipophilic, cross the blood-brain barrier rapidly and cause CNS depressant effect mediated through gamma-aminobutyric acid (GABA) agonism or NMDA receptor antagonism. In addition to CNS toxicity these substances also have significant toxicity to other body organs like liver and kidneys. Prolonged use may lead to neurocognitive disorders, anxiety and even psychosis. Use of inhalants can lead to serious medical complications such as cardiac arrhythmias and seizures. Sudden heavy sniffing may lead to death due to asphyxiation. Intoxication syndrome includes euphoria, excitation, disinhibition, slurred speech, memory impairment and delirium and coma with high doses. Sudden discontinuation of inhalants may lead to a withdrawal syndrome similar to alcohol. However benzodiazepines, other CNS depressants and adrenergic drugs should be avoided. Psychosocial interventions are valuable.

Keywords: Asphyxiation, Choking, Cleaning fluids, Deodorant spray, GABA, Gases, Gasoline, Glues, Hair sprays, Nail polish remover, Neurotoxicity, Nitrites, NMDA, Spray paints, Volatile hydrocarbons.

* **Corresponding author Subhash C. Bhatia:** Department of Psychiatry, Mental Health and Behavioral Sciences, Creighton University; Department VA Nebraska- Western Iowa Health Care System 4101 Woolworth Ave Omaha, NE 68105, USA; Tel/Fax: 402-9954315/402-995-4240; Email: sub55@cox.net

Subhash C. Bhatia (Ed.)

KEY LEARNING POINTS

1. Inhalants are volatile hydrocarbon-based substances when inhaled in a vapor form produce intoxication and pleasurable effect.
2. Inhalants are aerosols or volatile solvents like glues, gases, spray paints, nail polish remover, hair sprays, deodorants, gasoline, cleaning fluids, and nitrites. These don't include drugs that are sniffed or inhaled after burning like cannabis.
3. Most inhalants are central nervous system (CNS) depressants and can cause serious harm to vital organs including liver, heart, kidneys and brain.
4. Inhalants cause rapid high with excitation followed by drowsiness, disinhibition, light headedness and agitation. High amounts can produce confusion, delirium, anesthesia and loss of consciousness.
5. The effects may include diplopia, memory impairment, slurred speech, cardiac arrhythmias "sudden sniffing death" or death by asphyxiation, suffocation, seizures, coma, choking or motor vehicle accident.
6. Neurotoxic effects due to prolonged use may range from mild cognitive impairment to dementia.

CLINICAL VIGNETTE

A 14 year old male was brought to the emergency room (ER) by the ambulance. The patient was found unconscious by his mother with a rag soaked with gasoline in his hand. Pants and Underwear soaking wet, and smell like urine. On arrival at the emergency room he was confused and disoriented, with a gasoline odor on his breath. Examination also showed conjunctival injections, bilateral basal rales on auscultation, nystagmus, psychomotor retardation and Pulse: 53/Min. Complete blood count showed moderate leukocytosis and normocytic anemia, arterial blood gases showed mild hypercarbia.

DISCUSSION OF THE VIGNETTE

The vignette demonstrates a clinical history suggestive of acute intoxication with gasoline, with neurologic, cardiac and pulmonary symptoms. Some of the neurologic symptoms and signs resembled alcohol intoxication. Patient was placed in a low stimulation environment. Most symptoms resolved within 2 hours with supportive interventions.

DIAGNOSTIC CONSIDERATIONS

The diagnostic criteria listed in DSM-5 for inhalant-related disorder are: presence of two out of 10 symptoms during 12 months period. These include use of large quantities inhalant use for more than intended period, tolerance, craving and inability to cut down their use, compulsive use despite health consequences, large amount of time spent to acquire or recover from their effects and as a result failure to meet social, occupational, recreational or role obligations. Specifiers include type of inhalant used, early or sustained remission [1]. With long-term use a withdrawal syndrome characterized by irritability, anxiety, restlessness, insomnia and tremor may manifest. In DSM-5 Inhalant -Related disorders are listed, as Inhalants use disorder, Inhalants Intoxication, Other Inhalants-Induced disorders and Unspecified Inhalants use disorders. The diagnosis is generally by history. Breath saliva or urine may aid in diagnosis of inhalant use or non-inhalant substance use disorder.

EPIDEMIOLOGY

Children and adolescents between 12-17 living in poverty, homelessness and from an ethnic minority are at higher risk. Inhalants are important gateway drug. 2011 Monitoring the Future (MTF) survey of 8th, 10th and 12th graders revealed that 31.1 percent of 8th-graders have used inhalants in current or past-year [2]. According to 2010 National Survey on Drug Use and Health (NSDUH) 793,000 individuals aged 12 and older used inhalants for the first time during the last 12 months; 68.4 percent were under the age of 18 [3]. The inhalant use disorder frequently remits after adolescence and therefore significantly declines after age 20.

CLINICAL PSYCHOPHARMACOLOGY

There are thousands of inhalant compounds that are easily accessible and legal to obtain for industrial and house hold uses. These products include adhesives, aerosols, solvents, paint thinners, degreasers, lighter fluids, Freon, hair and paint sprays, computer dust cleaners, anesthetics, gasoline, laughing gas and nitrites *etc.* Inhalants are central nervous system (CNS) depressants. The mechanism of action of inhalants is not very well understood. Inhalants are rapidly absorbed in the lungs. Inhalant hydrocarbons are highly lipophilic and easily cross the blood brain barrier. Due to brain being lipid rich these also accumulate in the brain. Some inhalants like toluene are metabolized in the liver and others are exhaled in an unaltered form. Anesthetic gases such as nitrous oxide are N-methyl-D-aspartate (NMDA) receptor antagonists. Animal research shows that that CNS depressant effect may be mediated through gama-aminobutyric acid (GABA) agonism and or NMDA receptor antagonism [4]. In animal research toluene increases dopamine in nucleus accumbens, frontal cortex by stimulating area, thus leading to the reinforcing effect [5 - 7].

MEDICAL AND PSYCHIATRIC CONSEQUENCES OF INHALANT USE DISORDERS

Inhalants are highly toxic especially to lipid rich organ systems like the brain. Different inhalants may have some variation in presentation. Serious medical Complications include :

Chemical or aspiration pneumonia, cardiac failure or arrest, "sudden sniffing death" or death by asphyxiation, suffocation, seizures, coma, motor vehicle accidents due to lack of coordination [8]. Inhalant–induced cerebral damage and persistent dementia can be one of the outcomes of persistent and prolonged use. Other nervous system complications include: vision, hearing, and movement abnormalities due to sensory neural loss, loss of coordination, ataxia, and peripheral neuropathy, chlorinated hydrocarbons are associated with chemical hepatitis and liver damage, rhabdomyolysis and polyneuropathy. Liver and kidney damage may occur.

Inhalant abuse during pregnancy, using animal models, poses a developmental harm to fetus. This may result in reduced birth weights, skeletal abnormalities, neurobehavioral developmental delays and altered metabolism [9].

Nitrites are mainly abused by older adolescents and adults primarily to enhance sexual desire, performance and pleasure. This may be associated with unsafe sex and contracting or spreading infectious diseases like HIV /AIDS, hepatitis B and C. Nitrites are also reported to impair the immune system and increase the risk of infectious diseases like tuberculosis [10].

Inhalant-induced anxiety, mood and psychotic disorders are reported when the patient is not intoxicated, in withdrawal or in delirium.

PHARMACOLOGICAL INTERVENTIONS

Care of inhalant-intoxicated patient is primarily supportive.

There is no FDA approved treatment for inhalant use disorders. If a patient presents with anxiety, mood or psychotic disorders the role of pharmacotherapy is mostly symptomatic. Benzodiazepines should be avoided because they may enhance the depressant effect of inhalants. Also adrenergic drugs should also be avoided due to the risk of cardiac arrhythmia. Psychotic symptoms can improve with carbamazepine or haloperidol. However, carbamazepine will cause fewer extrapyramidal side effects [11].

Psychosocial Interventions

There is no specific research on the effectiveness of psychosocial interventions in inhalant use disorder. Most of those who are dependent on inhalants are also addicted to other substances. Therefore, motivational interviewing, cognitive-behavioral therapy and contingency management. Family therapy and engaging loved ones in the treatment can be of value.

Patients with suicidal intent, plan or attempt should he hospitalized in a psychiatric facility. Patients with severe cognitive and psychical impairments may require assisted living environments.

SUMMARY

Inhalant use disorders is a serious health condition with serious medical, including death, psychiatric and cognitive consequences. Unfortunately most users are children and adolescents between 12-17. Other demographic characteristics include poverty, homelessness and ethnic minority background. Educational programs for school aged children may be helpful. Supportive care and other biopsychosocial interventions used for other substance use disorder may also benefit these patients.

INHALANT USE DISORDER- PATIENT EDUCATION SHEET

What are Inhalants?

Inhalants are volatile chemical substances which produce vapors like glues, aerosols, solvents, paint thinners, degreasers, lighter fluids, Freon, hair and paint sprays, computer dust cleaners, anesthetics, gasoline, laughing gas and nitrites *etc*.

How are Inhalants Used?

Inhalants are breathed through nose or mouth by "sniffing", "snorting", spraying the aerosols directly in to mouth or nose, "bagging"- inhaling substance sprayed in to plastic or paper bag, "huffing" from an inhalant soaked rag stuffed in the mouth or inhaling from a balloon filled with nitrous oxide.

What Is Inhalants Use Disorder?

Inhalant abuse is the deliberate inhalation by "sniffing" or "huffing" fumes, vapors, or gases from common household commercial products such as gasoline for the purpose of "getting high" and using it again to experience that high .

Are Inhalants Addictive?

Yes. Inhalants are addictive because like other drugs these affect the reward circuits in the brain to cause "high". Repeated highs are the cause of addiction.

What are the Withdrawal Effects of Inhalants?

The withdrawal symptoms are: nervousness, irritability, disordered attention and concentration, restlessness, insomnia, disturbing dreams and tremor.

What Medical Complications can be Caused by Inhalants?

Inhalants may cause sudden death called "sudden sniffing death". In addition these can cause brain, liver and kidney damage, hearing and vision loss In addition there is increase risk of sexually transmitted diseases, HIV/AIDs, Hepatitis B and C. Brain damage may even cause dementia requiring nursing home placement.

What is "Sudden Sniffing Death" Mentioned Above?

It is a condition associated with cardiac arrest due to the use of inhalants any particularly air conditioning coolant (Freon), butane, propane, electronic contact cleaner and chemicals in some aerosol products.

Where can I Get More Information about Inhalants and Inhalant Related Disorders?

http://www.inhalant.org; www.drugabuse.gov

CONFLICT OF INTEREST

The authors confirm that they have no conflict of interest to declare for this publication.

ACKNOWLEDGEMENTS

Declared none.

REFERENCES

[1] Diagnostic and Statistical Manual of Mental Disorders. 5th ed., Arlington, VA: American Psychiatric Association 2013.

[2] Institute of Social Research. Monitoring the Future, 2011 (Study Results). Ann Arbor, MI: University of Michigan 2012. http://www.monitoringthefuture.org

[3] Office of Applied Studies: Results from 2010 National Survey on Drug Use and Health: Summary of National Findings HHS Pub No (SMA) 11-4658. Rockville, MD: SAMHSA 2011.

[4] Balster RL. Neural basis of inhalant abuse. Drug Alcohol Depend 1998; 51(1-2): 207-14. [http://dx.doi.org/10.1016/S0376-8716(98)00078-7] [PMID: 9716942]

[5] Riegel AC, French ED. An electrophysiological analysis of rat ventral tegmental dopamine neuronal activity during acute toluene exposure. Pharmacol Toxicol 1999; 85(1): 37-43. [http://dx.doi.org/10.1111/j.1600-0773.1999.tb01061.x] [PMID: 10426162]

[6] Gerasimov MR, Schiffer WK, Marstellar D, Ferrieri R, Alexoff D, Dewey SL. Toluene inhalation produces regionally specific changes in extracellular dopamine. Drug Alcohol Depend 2002; 65(3):

243-51.
[http://dx.doi.org/10.1016/S0376-8716(01)00166-1] [PMID: 11841896]

[7] Riegel AC, Zapata A, Shippenberg TS, French ED. The abused inhalant toluene increases dopamine release in the nucleus accumbens by directly stimulating ventral tegmental area neurons. Neuropsychopharmacology 2007; 32(7): 1558-69.
[http://dx.doi.org/10.1038/sj.npp.1301273] [PMID: 17213847]

[8] Maxwell JC. Deaths related to the inhalation of volatile substances in Texas: 1988-1998. Am J Drug Alcohol Abuse 2001; 27(4): 689-97.
[http://dx.doi.org/10.1081/ADA-100107662] [PMID: 11727883]

[9] Bowen SE, Batis JC, Paez-Martinez N, Cruz SL. The last decade of solvent research in animal models of abuse: mechanistic and behavioral studies. Neurotoxicol Teratol 2006; 28(6): 636-47.
[http://dx.doi.org/10.1016/j.ntt.2006.09.005] [PMID: 17064879]

[10] Soderberg LS. Increased tumor growth in mice exposed to inhaled isobutyl nitrite. Toxicol let 1999; 104(1-2): 35-41.
[http://dx.doi.org/10.1016/S0378-4274(98)00228-8]

[11] Hernandez-Avila CA, Ortega-Soto HA, Jasso A, Hasfura-Buenaga CA, Kranzler HR. Treatment of inhalant-induced psychotic disorder with carbamazepine *versus* haloperidol. Psychiatr Serv 1998; 49(6): 812-5.
[http://dx.doi.org/10.1176/ps.49.6.812] [PMID: 9634163]

CHAPTER 14

Opioid Use and Addictive Disorder

Teri Gabel[1,*], **Imad Alsakaf**[2] and **James Meyer**[3]

[1] *VA Nebraska Western Iowa Health Care System, Clinical Pharmacy Specialist - Mental Health, Omaha, NE 68105; Department of Psychiatry, University of Nebraska College of Medicine Omaha NE 68198; Drug Therapy Consultants, PC 5116 N 116 St, Omaha NE 68164 USA*

[2] *Creighton University School of Medicine 3528 Dodge Street Omaha, NE 68131 USA*

[3] *Inroads to Recovery 2808 N 75th ST Omaha NE, 68134 USA*

Abstract: This chapter discusses epidemiologic, pathophysiology and diagnostic issues associated with opioid use disorders. Differentiation of the recreational user and the user who was prescribed narcotics for a diagnosed pain issue is an important variable in the approach to management. Absolute sobriety from opiates/opioids is difficult to achieve and a multifaceted approach is a necessity. This chapter also describes non-drug therapies used in the management of opioid use disorders, including narcotics anonymous, cognitive behavioral therapies and others. For many patients, substitution therapy may be necessary for the short or long term to prevent further issues with opioid use and a better outcome. Buprenorphine substitution therapy requires special provider training while methadone must be dispensed by a licensed opiate treatment program. Withdrawal from opioids is not life threatening but is subjectively very distressing. Management of opioid withdrawal can include treatment with buprenorphine or methadone resulting in relief of withdrawal symptoms and then slowly tapering off the medication. Alternatively non-opiate agents such as clonidine and other medications for symptom relief are used to ameliorate withdrawal. The chapter includes key points and a case vignette to assist the learner. A patient education sheet and further resources are included.

* **Corresponding author Teri Gabel:** VA Nebraska Western Iowa Health Care System, Clinical Pharmacy Specialist - Mental Health, Omaha, NE 68105; Department of Psychiatry, University of Nebraska College of Medicine Omaha NE 68198; Drug Therapy Consultants, PC 5116 N 116 St, Omaha NE 68164 USA; Tel: (402)493-5222; Email: pharmdherb@gmail.com

Subhash C. Bhatia (Ed.)

Keywords: Buprenorphine, Clonidine, Methadone, Naloxone, Naltrexone, Suboxone, Substitution therapy, Subutex.

KEY LEARNING POINTS

1. The natural opiate products are morphine and codeine. These are made from opium which is extracted from the poppy plant.
2. Synthetic opioids include, heroin, hydromorphone, oxycodone, hydrocodone, meperidine, methadone and fentanyl.
3. Withdrawal from opioids is not dangerous but is subjectively very distressing.
4. Absolute sobriety from these drugs is rather difficult to achieve. Relapse is common, expect it, then get the patient back on the path to recovery.
5. Treatment of opioid use disorder is multifaceted. Treatment of comorbid psychiatric disorder(s) improves outcome.
6. Substitution therapy with buprenorphine or methadone or narcotic antagonist therapy is often required for a better outcome.

CLINICAL VIGNETTE

Sharon, a thirty-four year old married, ill-appearing white female, presents to your office stating that she is having a problem with her "pain pills." On further questioning, she provides the following information. She has been overusing the oxycodone (Oxycontin) that she has been getting for her chronic back pain. She says she is not even sure how much her back really hurts any more. She will also use hydrocodone (Vicodin) and oxycodone and acetaminophen (Percocet) because they are easier to get and she doesn't get questioned about these very often, but she worries about the acetaminophen content of these and possible liver damage. She prefers Oxycontin when she can get it, but finds it harder to obtain. She has gone to several different doctors and filled prescriptions at several different pharmacies so as to not raise any questions or arouse suspicion. She has friends that can help her get these medications on the street as well, and acknowledges that she has been doing this more over the past few months, at considerable expense. She has used as many as ten 80mg Oxycontin pills in a day. Most recently, she has been crushing these and snorting the powder to get a more immediate effect, instead of taking them orally. She reluctantly admits she has also tried intravenous use after a couple of friends encouraged her to try this and showed her how to prepare and inject it. She then states "And I'm not very good at it" as she exposes her left anterior forearm to show you multiple infected injection sites and needle tracks.

Sharon provides the following history: She grew up with both parents, a brother and sister with no family history of drug or alcohol problems. She did very well in school and graduated from high school at age eighteen. She received an athletic scholarship to attend college and play volleyball. She went to college and majored in social work. She played volleyball for all four years and did well. She hurt her back in her third year however, and this lead to her first use of opioids. She was provided Vicodin and took this so she could continue to play even when her back hurt. She graduated and married when she was twenty-three. Her husband is three years older and is a civil engineer. They now have three children, ages 5, 9, and 10. Her husband is quite successful and as a result she has not had to work. Her husband is aware of the patient's problems, though probably not to the complete extent or the severity. She feels her husband is probably losing patience with her. She has tried to quit on several occasions. Her use has varied over the past years with rapid escalation over the past two years. She acknowledged some limited marijuana use while in college but has had no use since. Her alcohol use has been moderate since her late teens. She has been very active socially with her own and her husband's friends and families. She stated she usually works out in a gym daily where she has met her "using" friends. On examination, Sharon says she is "withdrawing", and feeling "sick" having not used any opioids for over eighteen hours. She says she wants help in quitting so she can get things together and "save my marriage and life". She stated "I love my family and this is no way to live". She stated she hurts all over, she is nauseous and has diarrhea. Her vital signs are blood pressure 155/95, pulse 105, respiratory rate 22 and body temperature 100.6F.

Sharon's opioid withdrawal is anticipated to worsen, but of immediate concern was the left forearm. CBC showed markedly elevated WBC. One abscess required incision and drainage. Culture showed the bacterial agent to be Methicillin Resistant Staphylococcus Aureus (MRSA). Sharon was hospitalized and treated with IV vancomycin. Opioid withdrawal was managed with clonidine 0.1 mg twice daily and symptomatic therapy.

Because there is no Opiate Treatment Program (OTP) or a provider registered to prescribe buprenorphine the patient was discharged on naltrexone 50mg daily. Her treatment recommendations included birth control measures, scheduled and unscheduled urine drug screens, attendance at narcotic anonymous (NA) meetings and follow up with current provider.

EPIDEMIOLOGY

According to the Diagnostic and Statistical Manual of Mental Disorders, 5th edition [1], the 12-month prevalence of opioid use disorder in the community population for individuals ages 18 and older is 0.37%. This may be an underestimate because of the large number of individuals with opioid use disorders that are incarcerated. Rates are higher in males than females (0.49% *vs.* 0.26%), with the male to female ratio being 1.5:1 for opioids; for heroin it is 3:1. Female adolescents may have a higher likelihood of developing opioid use disorders. The prevalence rate decreases with age *i.e.* 0.82% among adults age 29 years or younger and 0.09% among adults age 65 years and older. Among adults, the prevalence rate of opioid use disorder is lower among African Americans at 0.18% but higher in Native Americans at 1.25%. It is close to average among whites (0.38%), Asian or Pacific Islanders (0.35%), and Hispanics (0.39%). In the USA, in the adolescent population ages 12-17yrs, the 2-month prevalence of opioid use disorder in a community population is approximately 1%, but the prevalence of heroin use disorder is less than 0.1%. Also, the prevalence rate of analgesic use disorder in adolescents 12-17 years is about 1%. In European countries, the 12-month prevalence rate of problematic opioid use in the community population ages 15-64 years is between 0.1% and 0.8%. The average prevalence rate of problematic opioid use in the European Union and Norway is between 0.36% and 0.44% [1].

Results from the National Epidemiologic Survey on Alcohol and Related Conditions (NESARC) indicate that the twelve-month and lifetime prevalence of the DSM-IV opioid abuse are 0.2 percent and 1.1 percent respectively and that the twelve-month and lifetime prevalence of DSM-IV opioid dependence are 0.1

percent and 0.3 percent respectively [2]. However, the lifetime prevalence of non-medical use of opioids was reported as 4.7 percent [3]. According to the National Survey on Drug Use and Health (NSDUH) in 2002, there were an estimated 600,000 individuals aged twelve or older in the United States who used heroin in the past year; about one third of these (210,000 individuals) met criteria for past-year DSM-IV dependence or abuse of heroin. However, heroin use is less prevalent than non-medical use of prescription opioids [4]. According to data from NSDUH, approximately 1.5 million persons aged 12 or older met the criteria for past-year DSM-IV abuse of or dependence on prescription pain relievers, second only to the rate for DSM-IV marijuana abuse or dependence (4.3 million) [4]. Since 1990, there has been a dramatic increase in the use and abuse of prescription narcotic analgesics in the United States, especially in rural communities [5].

Co-occurring Psychiatric and other Substance Use Disorder(s)

Findings from the NESARC study indicate that among all those who met the criteria for either lifetime DSM-IV opioid abuse or lifetime opioid dependence (578 individuals out of the total sample of 43093), about 70 percent met criteria for at least one non-substance use disorder Axis I diagnosis, 60 percent had at least one mood disorder, and 39 percent had at least one anxiety disorder. The most prevalent disorder was major depression, in over half (52 percent) of the sample. In addition about 50 percent met criteria for at least one personality disorder. The prevalence of antisocial personality disorder alone was 30 percent. In addition 22.6 percent and 70 percent met criteria for substance abuse or dependence on another substance respectively. Sixty-three percent and 22 percent met DSM-IV criteria for alcohol dependence and alcohol abuse respectively. Fifty percent had a history of marijuana abuse. One third had a history of cocaine, sedatives, amphetamines, hallucinogens, or tranquilizers abuse; and 11 percent inhalant abuse [4].

Of note is that women had twice the likelihood as men for having a lifetime mood disorder, and except for hypomanic disorder they were twice as likely as men to have each of the specific mood disorders. Also, they had nearly twice the probability as men for having an anxiety disorder except for panic disorder with or without agoraphobia. Overall, there was no significant gender difference in having any DSM-IV Axis I (non-substance use) disorder [3]. In comparison to men, women had about twice the odds of having paranoid personality disorder, but somewhat more than half as likely as men to have antisocial personality disorder.

A recent study has indicated that cyclothymic, and to a lesser extent irritable traits could represent the temperamental profile of heroin addicts, irrespective of co-morbidity and previous conceptual hypothesis of "sensation-seeking" and "novelty-seeking" as the main personality characteristics of addiction [5, 6]. About 15 percent of patients with opioid dependence attempt suicide at least once.

Co-occurring Medical Disorders

Potential consequences of intravenous drug use and sharing needles include HIV infection, Hepatitis B and C, endocarditis as well as other infectious diseases that might be systemic or localized to the skin and injection sites [7]. Persons might experience idiosyncratic allergic reactions to opioids which might result in anaphylactic shock, pulmonary edema and death [7]. In the context of opioid overdose an individual may experience respiratory depression, hypotension, bradycardia and hypothermia which might result in death [7]. About 75 percent of infants born to addicted mothers experience opioid withdrawal syndrome [7].

DIAGNOSIS AND CLINICAL PRESENTATION [7]

The euphoric effect of opioids leads to their repeated use and opioid use disorders. A common clinical situation involves a patient with unexplained physical pain such as headaches, back pain or abdominal pain being prescribed opioids, who then experiences the euphoric effects along with pain relief. This may lead to long-term continuation of opioids where it is no longer indicated. Drug-seeking behaviors subsequently follows, taking opioids in doses more than prescribed, filling prescriptions earlier or filling at multiple pharmacies to avoid detection.

The diagnosis of opioid use disorder can be challenging when the patient conceals past patterns of opioid use or is seeking the drug by exaggerating the degree of pain experienced.

The euphoric effect occurs with acute intoxication and is often described as a rush or similar to 'sexual orgasm'. The rush can last for several minutes and is followed by sedation which can last for several hours. Patients typically experience apathy after the rush. Other signs and symptoms of opioid intoxication include: pupillary constriction (or pupillary dilation from severe anoxia in overdose), impaired judgment, impairment in attention or memory, and slurred speech. Patients who take opioids over a long period of time will develop tolerance, characterized by decreasing effects of the drug over time, or the need for higher doses to achieve the same effect. Tolerance with intravenous heroin develops rapidly. Chronic use, if suddenly discontinued, leads to withdrawal symptoms, which indicates the presence of physical dependence. Heroin users, who are in an advanced stage of abuse, shift between euphoria and withdrawal symptoms several times in the course of a day. The euphoric effect of heroin is often potentiated by combining it with drugs like cocaine.

The rapid induction of tolerance and consequent drug-seeking behavior can lead to significant psychosocial consequences, including disruption in work, school and family obligations, crime, financial consequences and homelessness. More subtle is the impact on those with ready access to opioids, such as health care workers, until drug abuse leads to detection of diversion or work disruption.

Opioid withdrawal symptoms are easy to detect and occur after discontinuation or reduction in heavy or prolonged use. Symptoms begin within 6-8 hours after last drug intake. Typical symptoms are dysphoric mood, nausea or vomiting, muscle aches, lacrimation, rhinorrhea, pupillary dilation, piloerection, diarrhea, sweating, yawning, fever and insomnia. These autonomic symptoms result from the sudden withdrawal of opioid suppression of the noradrenergic locus ceruleus. Hence the benefits of α-2 adrenergic agonists like clonidine in relieving several opioid withdrawal symptoms. Opioid withdrawal is not life-threatening, though subjectively very distressing.

Opioid Related Disorders

The DSM-5 lists the following opioid related disorders [1]: Opioid Use Disorder, Opioid Intoxication, Opioid Withdrawal, Other Opioid-Induced Disorders, and

Unspecified Opioid-Related Disorders.

Opioid Use Disorder is characterized by problematic use with impairment. Details of the diagnostic criteria and Specifiers are listed in DSM-5 [1]. Symptoms include taking opioids in larger quantities than intended, desire to quit with unsuccessful attempts to do so, a lot of time utilized to use or recover from use, craving to reuse, use despite negative social, occupational, school or health consequences, tolerance and withdrawal.

Other Opioid-Induced Disorders, include Opioid Intoxication and Opioid Withdrawl and these symptoms are described above. Patients may also experience opioid intoxication and withdrawal delirium, opioid induced depressive and/or anxiety disorders, sleep disorders and sexual dysfunction [1].

Unspecified Opioid-Related Disorder, includes opioid use which does not meet any of the specific diagnostic criteria but still causes impairment or distress [1].

NEUROBIOLOGY OF OPIOID USE DISORDERS

The neurobiology of opioid use and induced disorders is complex. Opioid use disorders are chronic relapsing illnesses characterized by compulsive use despite negative consequences, intense craving amongst other factors precipitated by environmental cues. The repeated use is motivated by both experiencing pleasurable/rewarding effects and the desire to avoid the aversive effects of drug withdrawal [8, 9].

Opioid self-administration mimics the binding action of endogenous opioid peptides - endorphins, enkephalin and dynorphins respectively to mu, delta and kappa opioid receptors. The reinforcing effects of opioids is through binding activity at mu and delta receptors where as binding action at kappa receptors reduces the immediate rewarding effect of opiates [10].

The neural basis of opioid use disorders primarily points towards mesolimbic dopamine projections from the ventral tegmental area (VTA) to the nucleus accumbens (NAc) [11]. The mu opioid receptor agonists, like morphine, activate mesolimbic dopamine (DA) projections from the VTA. DA release in the NAc causes the euphoria/rewarding effect of morphine. In addition, mu receptor activation results in analgesia, nausea, reduced bowel motility, miosis (constricted pupils), sedation, reduced blood pressure and decreased respiration. With continued use, tolerance develops for sedation, euphoria and decreased respiration. To experience the same level of euphoria, often a higher dose of opioids is required. This forms the basis for tolerance. Little tolerance develops for analgesia, miosis and reduced bowel motility [12].

Delta opioid receptor activation produces analgesia but less than mu opioid receptor agonists. Also, evidence for respiratory depression is mixed. Delta opioid receptor agonists, however, show robust antidepressant effect and are being researched as a novel class of antidepressants [13].

Kappa opioid receptor agonists can cause dysphoria and aversive effects on opiate use and thereby may have potential role in remission [14, 15].

Chronic opioid use leads to neuroadaptation, such as a decrease in DA transmission from the VTA to the NAc (9) [16]. This may be the cause of dysphoria and craving in the early phase of withdrawal leading to reuse. Chronic use is also associated with neuroadaptation of other neurotransmitter systems. Amongst them is corticotrophin releasing factor (CRF) [17]. This may explain the role of stress and emotional states in craving and compulsive drug use mediated by effects on DA and endogenous opioid peptides [17].

The neurobiology of the association between environmental cues and drug seeking behavior reflects the ability of opioid drugs to modulate preexisting brain reinforcement mechanisms [18].

BIO-PSYCHO-SOCIAL TREATMENT

Mutual-help, peer-support group-counseling [19] is by far the most accessible form of treatment for substance abuse in the United States. Alcoholics Anonymous (AA), Narcotics Anonymous (NA) and other self help programs based on the 12 step model are the most readily available. Some of the others with different philosophies include Life Ring Secular Recovery, Self-Management and Recovery Training (SMART), and Women for Sobriety.

The effectiveness of NA and other 12 step programs as a subject has been difficult to study due to difficulty with randomization, and, when studied, the outcomes were not consistent [19]. A Cochrane Review of eight studies, published between 1967 and 2005, measuring the effectiveness of AA, found no significant difference between the results of AA and twelve-step facilitation approaches compared to other treatments [20]. It was suggested that AA's effectiveness may not be due to its specific content or process, rather, its chief strength may lie in its ability to provide free, long-term, easy access treatment and exposure to recovery-related common therapeutic elements with the dose of treatment being mainly controlled by the patient according to his/her perception of needs [22].

Traditional aspects of cognitive behavioral therapy including identifying automatic thoughts, core beliefs and working on cognitive restructuring are applicable in the substance abuse context. Examples of common high-risk cognitions include: “I need the drug to relax”, “I won't be funny if I am clean and sober”, and “Just one time won't hurt” [21, 23].

The coping-skills training approach does not attempt to reduce the impact of triggers. Rather, it accepts triggers as a given and seeks to train alternative responses to them, so that a person will have several ways of coping with the occurrence of a trigger situation in place of drinking/drug use [23]. Social Skills Training on the other hand focuses on addressing concrete areas and problems such as drink or drug refusal. Refusing requests for use, handling criticism, handling intimate relationships and enhancing social support networks [23] and relapse prevention are other important aspects of the behavioral interventions.

The first 3 months after initial treatment for substance disorders represent over a 50 percent risk of relapse. The intervention during this period should target situations that may be of high risk for relapse through helping patients anticipate and avoid decisions that may lead to that outcome; reviewing the patients' lifestyle and activities that are high-risk for relapse and fostering development of activities that are incompatible with drinking/drug use. Developing the patients' awareness of what high-risk situations tend to promote use, and ongoing alertness and attention to the situations in which they find themselves, as well as monitoring of their thoughts and feelings, to detect warning signs of impending risk as early as possible [23]. Several studies have shown that cognitive behavioral therapy interventions are an effective way to achieve abstinence and prevent relapse in alcohol, however, at this point there seems no clear evidence about its superiority to other psychosocial interventions [24].

Contingency Management (CM) is where desired behaviors are rewarded and undesired behaviors are negatively reinforced. Rewards like an increase in methadone dose, allowing take home doses, money, bus tickets, *etc.* are contingent on urine drug screens, with an immediate reinforcement schedule, are particularly effective [25].

Despite the scarcity of research, the existing evidence suggests that case management may improve psychosocial functioning, increase retention in treatment, and decrease relapse [25].

PHARMACOLOGICAL TREATMENT OF OPIOID USE DISORDERS

The terms opioids, opiates and narcotics are used and describe a group of pain medications of natural and synthetic origin. The natural products, morphine and codeine are made from opium extracted from the poppy plant. Synthetic medications include heroin, hydromorphone (Dilaudid), oxycodone (Percocet, Percodan, and Oxycontin), hydrocodone (Vicodin, Lorcet, and Lortab), meperidine (Demerol), methadone (Dolophine) and fentanyl (Duragesic).

Whether the patient has developed an opioid use disorder due to the appropriate use or the misuse of a narcotic prescription for pain or the illicit use of narcotic medications, the approach to treatment, pharmacologically, is the generally the similar.

Management of Acute Intoxication

Opioid overdose is a medical emergency. The antidote for opioid intoxication is naloxone (Narcan®). Naloxone is a pure opioid antagonist and competes with opioids at the mu, kappa and delta receptors. It displaces the opioid, and reverses the narcotic effect. In the absence of opioids, naloxone has little pharmacologic effect [26, 27].

Naloxone is administered intravenously. However, it can be administered intramuscularly or subcutaneously if necessary. The onset of effect changes when these alternative routes are used. Administered intramuscularly, the effect may be prolonged compared to the intravenous route; the onset of action may be slower when administered subcutaneously. Dosing for suspected or known opioid overdose is 0.4 to 2 mg intravenously, repeating every two to three minutes as needed. If the patient shows no response or improvement after 10 mg, the clinician may want to reconsider the diagnosis of opioid toxicity [28].

Studies indicate that patients who ingested longer acting opioids have a greater potential for a protracted period of intoxication. It is recommended to monitor the patient for a longer period of time and to consider a continuous infusion of naloxone at two-thirds of the initial bolus dose/hour [26].

Significant doses of naloxone may be required in cases of large overdoses and it can be administered without significant toxicity [28].

FDA Approved Agents for Detoxification and Maintenance Treatment

Three agents are FDA approved for the management of opioid use disorders. These are methadone, buprenorphine and naltrexone.

Methadone (Dolophine®, Methadose®)

Methadone is a synthetic opiate with full agonist activity at mu-opiate receptors and antagonistic action at N-methyl-D-aspartate (NMDA) receptors. It has a half-life of 8-59 hours and will accumulate with repeated doses with high individual variability (range 6-100+ hours) [35]. Methadone is metabolized in the liver by cytochrome isoenzymes (CYP 450) 3A4, 2B6 and 2D6; minor routes include 2C9, 2C19 and 1A2. It has moderate inhibitory activity for 2D6. Common side effects of methadone include the usual opioid effects, headache, excessive sweating and rash. More serious adverse reactions include extreme sedation, dizziness, hypoxia, hallucinations, severe confusion, tachycardia, swelling of hands and feet, warmth in the chest and shortness of breath. Methadone can prolong the QTc interval.

Methadone crosses the placenta and is rated FDA pregnancy risk category C. It is found only in very low amounts in breast milk and is considered to be of minimal risk during breast feeding [29].

Methadone carries a Black Box Warning regarding its use in the treatment of opioid detoxification or dependence - it can only be dispensed through a licensed Opiate Treatment Program (OTP). Patients registered with one OTP and cannot get their doses from another program without prior arrangements. During maintenance treatment, dosing of methadone occurs daily at the OTP and each dose of the medication is observed. After a certain amount of time, which varies according to state and federal laws, a patient can qualify to have take-home doses of medication [30].

In a 2002 report, the Substance Abuse and Mental Health Services Administration (SAMHSA) found that patients addicted to prescription pain medications require higher doses of methadone than other patients [31]. A recent meta-analysis of randomized controlled trials with methadone found that retention in OTPs increased when dosing was individualized and flexible. It also demonstrated that higher doses, when utilized appropriately, are associated with better retention [32].

Opioid dependent patients with chronic pain and the need for narcotic medication for pain management, may be prescribed methadone for both pain and dependence. When used in the management of pain there are no prescribing restrictions. However, it is important to identify that the treatment is for pain not purely dependence. When used in the management of pain methadone may be dosed two to three times a day.

Buprenorphine (Subutex®) and Buprenorphine and Naloxone (Suboxone®)

Buprenorphine is a mixed agonist/antagonist. It has partial agonist activity binding with very high affinity to the mu receptor with antagonist activity at the kappa-opioid receptor. Buprenorphine binds more strongly to opioid receptors in the brain than other opioids making it more difficult to achieve intoxication with other opioids and it can trigger withdrawal by blocking the effect of the other opioid at the receptor. The binding of buprenorphine at the mu receptor is approximately 30 times as potent as morphine [33].

Suboxone® contains the mu-opioid receptor antagonist naloxone at a ratio of 4/1 buprenorphine to naloxone. Naloxone's role is to block the effect of buprenorphine should the Suboxone be dissolved and injected intravenously.

Buprenorphine can be administered by intramuscular injection, intravenous infusion, a transdermal patch or as a sublingual tablet or film. It is not administered orally due to very high first pass metabolism through the liver. The wide array of delivery methods is reflective of its different uses. When used in the management of opioid addiction and dependence, the sublingual tablets or film are the approved dosage forms. Maximal effects of buprenorphine appear to occur in the 16-32mg dose range for sublingual tablets/film. Higher doses are unlikely to produce greater effects [33].

Buprenorphine is metabolized in the liver, by the CYP 450 3A4 isoenzyme, into norbuprenorphine which is then conjugated with glucuronic acid and eliminated primarily through excretion into the bile. The half-life of buprenorphine is 24-46 hours.

Prescription of buprenorphine products is restricted to physicians who have completed 8 hours of course work and have become waivered to prescribe buprenorphine. This approval is noted by an "X" DEA number. For more information on this process go to SAMHSA.gov.

The main side effect advantage of buprenorphine in comparison to other opiates is the minimal risk of causing respiratory depression. Because of its ceiling effect and poor bioavailability buprenorphine is safer in overdose than full opioid agonists. However, toxicity increases and fatalities have been reported in overdoses in combination with benzodiazepines and alcohol [34].

Buprenorphine can also be used in the management of pain but has not the dosing power to assist in the management of severe pain due to its ceiling effect. A buprenorphine waiver is still required when prescribed for pain.

Buprenorphine is not indicated for use in pregnancy, but practice guidelines recommend switching to Subutex® if the patient becomes pregnant while being treated with Suboxone® rather than discontinuing the medication.

Naltrexone

Naltrexone (Revia®, Depade®) is a pure opioid receptor antagonist blocking the binding of opiates to the opioid receptors and competitively displacing opiate molecules from these receptors. In contrast to naloxone, it is twice as potent, has a longer duration of action, and is effective when administered orally.

When initiating naltrexone the patient must be opioid free for seven to ten days. A naloxone or naltrexone challenge test should be administered to the patient prior to initiation of therapy if sobriety is in question. The initial dose is 25 mg a day and is increased to 50 mg daily if there are no signs of withdrawal following the initial dose. Naltrexone has a black box warning for hepatocellular injury when given in excessive doses and is contraindicated in patients with acute hepatitis or liver failure [35].

Success of naltrexone is highly reliant on adherence, patient motivation, as well as the patient's social and employment resources. A review of studies showed that oral naltrexone maintenance therapy in combination with psychosocial therapy is more efficacious in limiting heroin use during treatment than placebo in combination with psychosocial therapy. However, when naltrexone alone is compared to placebo, the results did not reach statistical significance. A statistically significant benefit was not found regarding retention in treatment, side effects or relapse at follow up. Limitations of the review include small study populations and lack of generalizability. The review concluded that a lack of evidence exists for the use of naltrexone in opioid dependence and more studies need to be done [33]. An update on oral naltrexone was performed by the same authors in 2011 with no further support for oral naltrexone being noted [36, 37].

Long-acting Injectable Naltrexone (Vivitrol®): A sustained release intramuscular injection (IM) was FDA approved for alcohol dependence in 2006 and for opioid dependency in 2010. The goal of the sustained release formulation is to offer the convenience of not having to take a pill on a daily basis but it can also address issues of non-adherence found with the oral, daily formulation [38, 39]. It has been demonstrated to be superior to placebo in assisting patients in maintaining sobriety and decreasing craving [39]. The disparity from the studies with oral naltrexone may reside in the enhanced adherence offered by the depot formulation.

Injection site reactions are the primary adverse reaction to injectable naltrexone. It is recommended that patients should monitor the injection site and contact their provider if they develop pain, swelling, tenderness, redness, induration, bruising, or itching at the site of the injection that lasts longer than two weeks or gets worse with time. It is recommended by the FDA that these patients be promptly referred to a surgeon.

It is suggested that the long-acting IM formulation may have a decreased risk of liver toxicity but more studies are needed to confirm this.

Patient education regarding the danger of using opiates while on naltrexone is absolutely necessary and a treatment contract is recommended. If a patient attempts to use his/ her previous opiate dose or more to override the effect of naltrexone this could result in a lethal overdose.

MANAGING DETOXIFICATION

Signs and symptoms associated with opioid withdrawal usually begin 6 to 12 hours after the last dose of an opiate, peaking within two to four days then fading out over 7-14 days. Due to the longer half-life of methadone, the signs and symptoms may not develop for over 36 hours after the last dose.

Acute withdrawal from opiates and opioid medications can be managed symptomatically using non-opioid or opioid medications to target the range of withdrawal symptoms experienced. As mentioned earlier, withdrawal is not life threatening but is very uncomfortable and depending on the half-life of the medication in question can be quite significant and protracted.

Medications used to manage withdrawal symptoms include clonidine and lofexidine (alpha2-adrenergic agonists) to handle the adrenergic symptoms such as shivering, gooseflesh, anxiety, and high blood pressure [40]. Data suggests that lofexidine may be better tolerated that clonidine. See Table **1** for dosing of the alpha-adrenergic agents. Anti-nausea medications, acetaminophen or ibuprofen for headache and muscle aches and pain; calcium, magnesium and muscle relaxants to prevent or treat muscle cramping can also increase the comfort of a patient going through withdrawal. Studies indicate the alpha-adrenergic agents are superior to placebo but less effective than methadone or buprenorphine for managing withdrawal symptoms [40, 41].

Table 1. Alpha-adrenergic medications - doses for opioid detoxification*.

<table>
<tr><th>Agent</th><th>Dose</th><th>Comments</th></tr>
<tr><td>Clonidine</td><td>0.1 to 0.2mg TID
Max: 1mg a day</td><td rowspan="2">Monitor blood pressure prior to each dose. Decrease or hold the dose if the pressure is too low.
Side Effects: low blood pressure, dizziness, dry mouth, lack of energy
Lofexidine has less of an effect on blood pressure</td></tr>
<tr><td>Lofexidine</td><td>0.4 to 0.6mg TID
Max: 2mg a day</td></tr>
</table>

*This use is off-label for both agents.

The narcotic agents available for managing withdrawal include methadone and buprenorphine. Use of these agents during acute withdrawal eliminates or at least minimizes withdrawal symptoms and once the symptoms are managed a slow taper of the narcotic medication is initiated.

Treatment with methadone or buprenorphine (or buprenorphine and naloxone) is started at low doses given when the signs of withdrawal are present. The dose is then titrated over several days until the dose which eliminates withdrawal symptoms for a 24 hour period is attained. Some patients may require large doses of medication depending on their level of tolerance and the dose of opioid previously abused. In detoxification, the dose that eliminates the withdrawal symptoms is then slowly tapered. Breakthrough withdrawal symptoms can be addressed with the non-opioid medications mentioned previously.

MAINTENANCE TREATMENT

The goal of methadone and buprenorphine in the medical management of opioid dependence during maintenance treatment is to decrease or negate euphoria from the use of other opiates and to prevent the development of withdrawal symptoms. The dose that suppresses opioid withdrawal symptoms for a 24 hour period is generally the maintenance dose although this may need to be adjusted initially. Over time maintenance doses trend downward to the lowest necessary dose to maintain patient comfort.

Monitoring the Patient on Methadone and Buprenorphine [42]

Methadone and buprenorphine require special circumstances for their prescription in the management of opioid use disorder. This may limit a primary care providers experience with these agents. However, as mentioned earlier, the use of methadone as analgesic does not require that the medication be given at an OTP. A baseline EKG as clinically indicated is recommended in patients with co-morbid cardiac disease.

The use of a narcotic contract can be a helpful tool in the management of a patient, with or without a history of opioid use disorder, requiring a narcotic medication for pain. The contract can assist with "what ifs". Everything is laid out in advance and the consequences well known at the beginning. Each contract should be patient specific. Urine drug screening can be a part of these contracts. Substance use disorders are relapsing and remitting disorders and a positive urine for an opiate in a sober individual, a different opiate than the prescribed one, or a positive test for a stimulant or marijuana or an illicit substance, may have a different consequence. Please see the chapter in this book on urine drug screens for more information.

A positive therapeutic alliance between the patient and their primary care provider can be a stong benefit to the patient striving to deal with opioid use disorders.

Clinical Vignette Resolution

Sharon is attending NA and has obtained and retained a sponsor. Her urine drug screens have been negative. She has difficulty remembering to take the daily naltrexone doses. She also does not like to take pills because it reminds her of using narcotics. She requested to be started on the long-acting injectable formulation of naltrexone to assist with further sobriety.

SUMMARY

Management of opioid use disorders are challenging. Psycho-physiologic intolerance to discomfort and pain need to be addressed by both non-pharmacologic and pharmacologic interventions.

OPIOID USE DISORDER- PATIENT INFORMATION SHEET

What are Opioid use Disorders?

Opiate use disorders can result from the use of illicit heroin, the misuse of prescription narcotics or the correct use over time of prescription narcotics.

What are the Symptoms of Opioid Intoxication?

Opioids are abused for their euphoric, sedating and numbing effects. However, as tolerance develops the person requires larger doses for the positive effect and use needs to be maintained to prevent withdrawal symptoms.

With the use of high doses the person may become confused and have slurred speech. Small pupils are seen with intoxication as is respiratory depression – slow shallow breathing. Severe intoxication is a life-threatening situation.

What are the Common Symptoms of Opioid Withdrawal?

Persons who are dependent on opioids experience symptoms of withdrawal if they do not use frequently, including nervousness, anxiety, irritability, trouble concentrating, and agitation. Flu-like symptoms are common. Use of an opioid relieves these symptoms.

What Complications can Result from Opioid Dependence?

Legal consequences can be common if illicit substances are used or prescription medications are stolen. Anxiety and depression can result from opioid dependence and can be severe in some cases.

Death by overdose is unfortunately common. It is imperative that the patient understand that they can not use previous doses safely. After a few short weeks off of opiates the body resets as if it were opioid naive.

How is it Treated?

Medications

Options for treatment include detoxification and maintenance therapy.

Narcotic and non-narcotic medications can be used to offer symptomatic relief during withdrawal for detoxification.

Maintenance therapy options include methadone and buprenorphine. Methadone is only available for methadone maintenance through special treatment centers. Buprenorphine can be obtained from specially trained physicians.

Speak to your provider about sobriety and whether one of these medications might be an option or you.

Non-pharmacological Options

Support groups such as Narcotics Anonymous are available in most cities. Self-help materials are also available.

Resources

Narcotics Annonymous and other Support groups – community and online www.kap.samhsa.gov/products/brochures/pdfs/med_assisted_tx_facts.pdf

CONFLICT OF INTEREST

The authors confirm that they have no conflict of interest to declare for this publication.

ACKNOWLEDGEMENTS

Declared none.

REFERENCES

[1] Diagnostic and Statistical Manual of Mental Disorders. 5th ed., Arlington, VA: American Psychiatric Association 2013.

[2] Huang B, Dawson DA, Stinson FS, *et al.* Prevalence, correlates, and comorbidity of nonmedical prescription drug use and drug use disorders in the United States: Results of the National

Epidemiologic Survey on Alcohol and Related Conditions. J Clin Psychiatry 2006; 67(7): 1062-73. [http://dx.doi.org/10.4088/JCP.v67n0708] [PMID: 16889449]

[3] Grella CE, Karno MP, Warda US, Niv N, Moore AA. Gender and comorbidity among individuals with opioid use disorders in the NESARC study. Addict Behav 2009; 34(6-7): 498-504. [http://dx.doi.org/10.1016/j.addbeh.2009.01.002] [PMID: 19232832]

[4] Hall AJ, Logan JE, Toblin RL, *et al.* Patterns of abuse among unintentional pharmaceutical overdose fatalities. JAMA 2008; 300(22): 2613-20. [http://dx.doi.org/10.1001/jama.2008.802] [PMID: 19066381]

[5] Maremmani I, Pacini M, Popovic D, *et al.* Affective temperaments in heroin addiction. J Affect Disord 2009; 117(3): 186-92. [http://dx.doi.org/10.1016/j.jad.2009.01.007] [PMID: 19201034]

[6] Sadock BJ, Sadock VA, Eds. Synopsis of Psychiatry. 9th ed., Philadelphia: Lippincott Williams & Wilkins 2003.

[7] Sadock BJ, Sadock VA, Eds. Sadock Kaplan & Sadock's Comprehensive Textbook of Psychiatry Lippincott Williams & Wilkins. 7th ed., Philadelphia 2000.

[8] Wikler A. Recent progress in research on the neurophysiologic basis of morphine addiction. Am J Psychiatry 1948; 105(5): 329-38. [http://dx.doi.org/10.1176/ajp.105.5.329] [PMID: 18890902]

[9] Koob GF, Stinus L, Le Moal M, Bloom FE. Opponent process theory of motivation: neurobiological evidence from studies of opiate dependence. Neurosci Biobehav Rev 1989; 13(2-3): 135-40. [http://dx.doi.org/10.1016/S0149-7634(89)80022-3] [PMID: 2682399]

[10] Nestler EJ. Cellular and molecular mechanism of drug addiction. In: Charney DS, Nestler EJ, Eds. Neurobiology of mental illness. 2nd ed. New York: Oxford University Press 2004; pp. 698-709.

[11] Di Chiara G, Imperato A. Drugs abused by humans preferentially increase synaptic dopamine concentrations in the mesolimbic system of freely moving rats. Proc Natl Acad Sci USA 1988; 85(14): 5274-8. [http://dx.doi.org/10.1073/pnas.85.14.5274] [PMID: 2899326]

[12] Wikipedia contributors, . "M-opioid receptor," Wikipedia, The Free Encyclopedia Available from: https://en.wikipedia.org/w/index.php?title=%CE%9C-opioid_receptor&oldid=691720445 , [cited: 27th December 2009];

[13] Wikipedia contributors, . "Δ-opioid receptor," Wikipedia, The Free Encyclopedia Available from: https://en.wikipedia.org/w/index.php?title=%CE%94-opioid_receptor&oldid=696757358 , [cited: 27th December 2009];

[14] Wikipedia contributors, . "K-opioid receptor," Wikipedia, The Free Encyclopedia Available from: https://en.wikipedia.org/w/index.php?title=%CE%9A-opioid_receptor&oldid=696947206 , [cited: 27th December 2009];

[15] Xi ZX, Fuller SA, Stein EA. Dopamine release in the nucleus accumbens during heroin self-administration is modulated by kappa opioid receptors: an in vivo fast-cyclic voltammetry study. J Pharmacol Exp Ther 1998; 284(1): 151-61. [PMID: 9435173]

[16] Diana M, Pistis M, Carboni S, Gessa GL, Rossetti ZL. Profound decrement of mesolimbic dopaminergic neuronal activity during ethanol withdrawal syndrome in rats: electrophysiological and biochemical evidence. Proc Natl Acad Sci USA 1993; 90(17): 7966-9. [http://dx.doi.org/10.1073/pnas.90.17.7966] [PMID: 8367449]

[17] Sarnyai Z, Shaham Y, Heinrichs SC. The role of corticotropin-releasing factor in drug addiction. Pharmacol Rev 2001; 53(2): 209-43. [PMID: 11356984]

[18] Koob GF, Sanna PP, Bloom FE. Neuroscience of addiction. Neuron 1998; 21(3): 467-76. [http://dx.doi.org/10.1016/S0896-6273(00)80557-7] [PMID: 9768834]

[19] Wikipedia contributors, . "Alcoholics Anonymous," Wikipedia, The Free Encyclopedia Available from: https://en.wikipedia.org/w/index.php?title=Alcoholics_Anonymous&oldid=697524815 , [cited: 28th December 2009];

[20] Ferri M, Amato L, Davoli M. Alcoholics Anonymous and other 12-step programmes for alcohol dependence. Chochrane Database of Systematic Reviews 2006, Issue 3. Art. No. CD005032. doi. 2006;10:14651858 Available from: http://addictions-therapy.co.uk/pdf/Ferri_et_al.pdf , [cited: 30th December 2015];

[21] The Role of Nonpharmacologic Therapy in Alcohol Dependence: . Psychotherapy for Alcohol Dependence Available from: http://www.medscape.com/viewarticle/557742_4 , [cited: 28th December 2009];

[22] Kelly JF, Magill M, Stout RL. How do people recover from alcohol dependence? A systematic review of the research on mechanisms of behavior change in alcoholics anonymous. Addict Res Theory 2009; 17(3): 236-59. [http://dx.doi.org/10.1080/16066350902770458]

[23] Kadden RM. Cognitive-behavior therapy for substance dependence: . Coping skills training. Unpublished work. 2002 Available from: http://www.ci2i.research.va.gov/CI2IRESEARCH/docs/Cogbehtrpguidelines.pdf , [cited: 28th December 2009];

[24] Morgenstern J, Longabaugh R. Cognitive-behavioral treatment for alcohol dependence: a review of evidence for its hypothesized mechanisms of action. Addiction 2000; 95(10): 1475-90. [http://dx.doi.org/10.1046/j.1360-0443.2000.951014753.x] [PMID: 11070524]

[25] Gold PB, Brady KT. Evidenced-based treatments for substance abuse disorders. Focus 2003; 1: 115-22. [http://dx.doi.org/10.1176/foc.1.2.115]

[26] Clarke SF, Dargan PI, Jones AL. Naloxone in opioid poisoning: walking the tightrope. Emerg Med J 2005; 22(9): 612-6. [http://dx.doi.org/10.1136/emj.2003.009613] [PMID: 16113176]

[27] Naloxone. In: Clinical Pharmacology [database on the Internet] . Tampa (FL): Gold Standard; 2009 Available from: www.clinicalpharmacology.com , [cited 23rd December 2009]; Subscription required to view.

[28] Naloxone. In: MicroMedex Healthcare Series [database on the Internet] . Ann Arbor (MI): Truven Health Analytics; 2015 Available from: www.micromedexsolutions.com , [cited: 28th December

2009]; Subscription required to view.

[29] Methadone. In: Micromedex Healthcare Series [database on the Internet] . Ann Arbor (MI): Truven Health Analytics; 2015 Available from: www.micromedexsolutions.com , [cited: 28th December 2009]; Subscription required to view.

[30] Medication-Assisted Treatment for Opioid Addiction in Opioid Treatment Programs Treatment Improvement Protocol (TIP) Series 43 DHHS Publication No (SMA) 05-4048. Rockville, MD: Substance Abuse and Mental Health Services Administration 2005.

[31] Results from the 2002 National Survey on Drug Use and Health: National Findings NHSDA Series H-22, DHHS Publication No (SMA) 03-3836. Rockville, MD: Office of Applied Studies, SAMHSA 2003. c

[32] Bao YP, Liu ZM, Epstein DH, Du C, Shi J, Lu L. A meta-analysis of retention in methadone maintenance by dose and dosing strategy. Am J Drug Alcohol Abuse 2009; 35(1): 28-33. [http://dx.doi.org/10.1080/00952990802342899] [PMID: 19152203]

[33] Treatment Improvement Protocol (TIP) Series 40. DHHS Publication No. (SMA) 04-3939. Rockville, MD: Substance Abuse and Mental Health Services Administration, 2004. Available from: http://buprenorphine.samhsa.gov/Bup_Guidelines.pdf , [cited: 28th December 2009];

[34] Wikipedia contributors, . "Buprenorphine," Wikipedia, The Free Encyclopedia Available from: https://en.wikipedia.org/w/index.php?title=Buprenorphine&oldid=697084705 , [cited: 28th December 2009];

[35] Naltrexone. In: Micromedex Healthcare Series [database on the Internet]. Ann Arbor (MI): Truven Health Analytics; 2015 Available from: www.micromedexsolutions.comcited: 28th December 2009 Subscription required to view.

[36] Minozzi S, Amato L, Vecchi S, Davoli M, Kirchmayer U, Verster A. Oral naltrexone maintenance treatment for opioid dependence. Cochrane Database Syst Rev 2006; 25(1): CD001333. [review]. [PMID: 16437431]

[37] Minozzi S, Amato L, Vecchi S, Davoli M, Kirchmayer U, Verster A. Oral naltrexone maintenance treatment for opioid dependence. Cochrane Database Syst Rev 2011; 13(4): CD001333. [PMID: 21491383]

[38] Lobmaier P, Kornør H, Kunøe N, Bjørndal A. Sustained-release naltrexone for opioid dependence. Cochrane Database Syst Rev 2008; 2(2): CD006140. [review]. [PMID: 18425938]

[39] Krupitsky E, Nunes EV, Ling W, Illeperuma A, Gastfriend DR, Silverman BL. Injectable extended-release naltrexone for opioid dependence: a double-blind, placebo-controlled, multicentre randomised trial. Lancet 2011; 377(9776): 1506-13. [http://dx.doi.org/10.1016/S0140-6736(11)60358-9] [PMID: 21529928]

[40] Gerra G, Zaimovic A, Giusti F, *et al.* Lofexidine *versus* clonidine in rapid opiate detoxification. J Subst Abuse Treat 2001; 21(1): 11-7. [http://dx.doi.org/10.1016/S0740-5472(01)00178-7] [PMID: 11516922]

[41] Gowing L, Farrell M, Ali R, White JM. Alpha2-adrenergic agonists for the management of opioid withdrawal. Cochrane Database Syst Rev 2009; 2(2): CD002024.

[PMID: 19370574]

[42] Gitlow S. Opioid dependence. substance use disorders: a practical guide. 2nd ed. Philadelphia: Lippincott Williams & Wilkins 2006; pp. 182-4.

CHAPTER 15

Phencyclidine (PCP) Use Disorder

Subhash C. Bhatia[1,*] and **Aly Hassan**[2]

[1] *Department of Psychiatry, Mental Health and Behavioral Sciences, Creighton University; Department VA Nebraska- Western Iowa Health Care System 4101 Woolworth Ave Omaha, NE 68105, USA*

[2] *Phoenix VA Health Care System, Department of Psychiatry, University of Arizona, Phoenix College of Medicine, Gilbert VA Clinic, 3285 S Val Vista Drive, Gilbert AZ 85925, USA*

Abstract: PCP is highly lipophilic dissociative anesthetic and a hallucinogen. This has been available since early 1950s. Its recreational use started in 1960's. It is smoked, snorted or consumed orally. PCP works through NMDA receptor antagonism as well as through direct and indirect dopaminergic effects leading to psychosis. Intoxication with low to moderate dose produce numbness in the extremities, unsteady gait, slurred speech, bloodshot eyes, horizontal, vertical or rotator nystagmus, tachycardia, hypertension, elevation of body temperature, shallow breathing, dry skin, loss of balance, muscle rigidity, agitation, aggression false sense of invulnerability and superior strength leading to daring acts like jumping off of high building. A moderate dose may produce analgesia and anesthesia. High dose may cause drop in blood pressure, heart and respiratory rate, seizures, coma and death. The presence of nystagmus may assist in differentiating PCP psychosis from other causes of psychoses.. Long-term effects of PCP may include "flash-backs", similar to LSD, persistent speech problems, memory impairment, chronic anxiety, depression or psychosis. There is no specific PCP antagonist medication. Supportive care in an environment of reduced sensory stimulation, urine acidification, and sedation with benzodiazepines is recommended. For patients with psychosis antipsychotic medication may be warranted. Psychosocial interventions add significant value.

Keywords: Angel Dust, Dissociative Anesthetic, NMDA Receptor Antagonist, PCP, Phencyclidine, Psychotomimetic drug.

[*] **Corresponding author Subhash C. Bhatia:** Department of Psychiatry, Mental Health and Behavioral Sciences, Creighton University; Department VA Nebraska- Western Iowa Health Care System 4101 Woolworth Ave Omaha, NE 68105, USA; Tel/Fax: (402) 995-4315/(402) 995-4240; Email: sub55@cox.net

KEY LEARNING POINTS

1. Phencyclidine (PCP) also known as Angel Dust was introduced in the early fifties as a "dissociative anesthetic" because it causes detachment (dissociation) from the environment and self. Its recreational use started in the 60s.
2. Users may experience feelings of superior strength and invulnerability, a numbing effect on the mind and its use is often associated with psychomotor agitation and aggression.
3. Long-term users of PCP may report memory loss, depression, disturbances of speech and thinking and weight loss.
4. PCP is addictive. Its repeated use causes craving and compulsive PCP-seeking behavior. It may be ingested, injected intravenously, inhaled or smoked by lacing cannabis with it or by dipping a cigarette in a fluid containing PCP.
5. PCP is primarily an NMDA receptor antagonist, but is also a dopamine agonist and an analgesic through effects on endorphin and enkephalin opioid receptors.
6. Chronic PCP use is associated with the development of psychosis indistinguishable from schizophrenia, possibly because PCP is a dopamine-2 receptor partial agonist and an inhibitor of dopamine reuptake.

CLINICAL VIGNETTE

An elderly couple contacted the emergency service frantically asking for help because their young neighbor broke into their apartment. They reported that "the young man is angry and is not making sense". They locked themselves in their bedroom until the police arrived. The individual was restless and incoherent; he grabbed a kitchen knife and charged towards a policeman who in turn shot him in the chest, a sad but true story.

DISCUSSION OF VIGNETTE

This person did not present to our clinic but from the news paper reports it is clear that patients with PCP intoxication often display unpredictable, belligerent, and assaultive behaviors.

EPIDEMIOLOGY

In USA in 2007 nearly 6.1 million persons aged 12 or older reported that they had used PCP during their life time. Of these, 137,000 individuals used PCP in the last year. In 2006 50,000 more individuals in this age group used PCP, a rather unfavorable trend.

NEUROPSYCHOPHARMACOLOGY

PCP is classified as a dissociative anesthetic. It is an extremely lipid soluble substance and rapidly crosses the blood brain barrier. Most often the street dose of 5mg is consumed orally, by inhalation, smoking or even through topical application [1]. This dose results in a high enough serum concentration to manifest psychotic symptoms. Higher serum concentrations lead to unconsciousness and coma. The powder form of PCP is more popular. When the powder is sprinkled on marijuana, parsley, or mint and smoked or the powder is snorted, the effects are felt within 5 minutes and may last up to 6 hours [2]. PCP acts mainly through the antagonism of NMDA receptors similar to ketamine, another dissociate anesthetic. This hypoactivity of NMDA receptors may also contribute to psychosis [3]. PCP is also a partial agonist of D2 receptors as well as a dopamine reuptake blocker, these actions may be the reason for its psychotomimetic effects [4, 5]. In addition PCP acts on endorphin and enkephalin opioid receptors [6] a mechanism for its analgesic effects. PCP is known to cause tolerance and addiction. 10% of unaltered and 25-30% of conjugated metabolite of PCP is excreted in the urine and can be detected by urine test for up to 8 days [7]. Lamotrigine may cause false positive test.

PCP INTOXICATION

Low to moderate doses of PCP produce numbness in the extremities, intoxication characterized by an unsteady gait, slurred speech, bloodshot eyes, horizontal, vertical or rotator nystagmus, tachycardia, hypertension, elevation of body temperature, shallow breathing, dry skin, loss of balance, muscle rigidity, agitation and aggression. A moderate dose also produces analgesia and anesthesia. With high doses, blood pressure heart and respiratory rates drop. It may lead to seizures, coma and death often due to accidental injury or suicide. The presence of nystagmus may assist in differentiating PCP psychosis from other causes of psychoses

Psychological effects include psychomotor agitation, aggression, impulsive, unpredictable, assaultive behavior that may start during or soon after PCP use. Other dose related effects may include euphoria or dysphoria, calmness, or extreme anxiety, feelings of superior strength and invulnerability, lethargy, disorientation, loss of coordination, distinct changes in body awareness, distorted sensory perceptions, impaired concentration, disordered thinking, illusions and hallucinations, agitation, combativeness, violence, memory loss, bizarre behavior, sedation, and stupor and coma.

DSM-5 provides the diagnostic criteria for phencyclidine use disorder and phencyclidine intoxication [7].

TREATMENT OF PCP USE AND PCP INDUCED DISORDERS

Pharmacotherapy

There are no FDA approved therapies nor there is a specific PCP antagonist. Supportive care including reducing environmental sensory stimulation is the main stay of management.

For acute phencyclidine intoxication the goal of therapy is to mitigate behavioral symptoms due to intoxication by sedation, this will reduce psychomotor agitation, anxiety and, based on psychotropic drug administered, psychosis also. Benzodiazepines have been effective for sedation. Antipsychotic medications with low intrinsic anticholinergic side effects and a lesser tendency to lower the seizure threshold like haloperidol are valuable for the management of severe agitation and psychosis. In addition the low anticholinergic profile of haloperidol does not negatively affect body temperature. If psychosis persists in patients vulnerable to developing schizophrenia continued antipsychotic therapy will be needed. Rhabdomyolysis is potentially a very serious effect of PCP intoxication. Acidification of urine (with ammonium chloride or ascorbic acid) has been a common practice however evidence suggests that the risks exceed the benefits [8]. This may require a nephrology consult and dialysis.

Psychosocial Interventions

Cognitive behavioral therapy, social skills training, enhancing coping skills and self-help groups are recommended.

SUMMARY

PCP is a dissociative anesthetic and one of the hallucinogens. During intoxication it can provoke violence and even may cause death by drowning, leaping from a high building, motor vehicle and other accidents, self-mutilation and suicide. Long-term effects may include "flash-backs", similar to LSD, persistent speech problems, memory impairment, chronic anxiety or depression or psychosis.

PCP - PATIENT EDUCATION SHEET

What is PCP?

Phencyclidine or PCP, on the streets it is also called "Angel Dust", is one of the hallucinogens which was in the 50's used for anesthesia in humans. However due to its tendency to cause agitation, catatonia and psychosis during surgery, in 1965 it was withdrawn from human use. At present as a controlled substance it is only used for animals. It is available in tablet, powder of liquid form. Sometimes other substances like marijuana are laced with this.

What Can PCP do to a Person?

It can cause physical symptoms like an unsteady gait, slurred speech, bloodshot eyes, rapid heartbeat, elevation of blood pressure, elevation of body temperature, shallow breathing, dry skin, muscle stiffness even kidney failure; or psychological effects like agitation, aggression, impulsive unpredictable assaultive behavior, homicidal and suicidal tendencies, illusion, hallucinations, paranoia, memory loss, bizarre behavior, stupor, coma and death.

Is PCP Addictive?

Yes, PCP is addictive and individuals use the drug compulsively despite the negative consequences.

How is this Addiction Diagnosed?

About 10% of PCP is excreted in the urine unaltered and can be detected by a urine drug test for up to 8 days. In addition when the person is intoxicated physical and psychological evaluation can provide clues towards its use.

How is PCP Addiction Treated?

There is no approved drug for its treatment. Whatever symptom is seen is treated, for psychosis a major tranquilizer like Haldol (haloperidol) is prescribed. In terms of therapy cognitive behavioral therapy, social skills training, enhancing coping skills and self-help groups are recommended.

Where Can I Get More Information?

The following web site: http://www.nida.nih.gov/PDF/RRHalluc.pdf

CONFLICT OF INTEREST

The authors confirm that they have no conflict of interest to declare for this publication.

ACKNOWLEDGEMENTS

Declared none.

REFERENCES

[1] Burns RS, Lerner SE. Perspectives: acute phencyclidine intoxication. Clin Toxicol 1976; 9(4): 477-501.
[http://dx.doi.org/10.3109/15563657608988151] [PMID: 789004]

[2] NIDA, Recreational Drugs Information. N.D. PCP as a Recreational Drug. Available from: http://www.a1b2c3.com/drugs/pcp2.htm 2001.

[3] Stahl SM. Stahl's essential psychopharmacology: neuroscientific basis and practical applications. 4th ed., New York: Cambridge University Press 2013.

[4] Giannini AJ, Kalavsky S, Loiselle RH, Giannini MC, Price WA. Possible role of the DA-2 receptor in phencyclidine psychosis. Neuroscience Abstracts 1983; 9: 33.

[5] Seeman P, Guan HC, Hirbec H. Dopamine D2High receptors stimulated by phencyclidines, lysergic acid diethylamide, salvinorin A, and modafinil. Synapse 2009; 63(8): 698-704.
[http://dx.doi.org/10.1002/syn.20647] [PMID: 19391150]

[6] Castellani S, Giannini AJ, Adams PM. Effects of naloxone, metenkephalin, and morphine on phencyclidine-induced behavior in the rat. Psychopharmacology (Berl) 1982; 78(1): 76-80. [http://dx.doi.org/10.1007/BF00470593] [PMID: 6815700]

[7] Diagnostic and Statistical Manual of Mental Disorders. 5th ed., Arlington, VA: American Psychiatric Association 2013.

[8] Baldridge EB, Bessen HA. Phencyclidine. Emerg Med Clin North Am 1990; 8(3): 541-50. [PMID: 2201519]

CHAPTER 16

Sedative, Hypnotic or Anxiolytic-Related Disorders

Subhash C. Bhatia[1,2,*], **Shashi K. Bhatia**[3], **Venkata Kolli**[4] and **Jaya krishna Madabushi**[5]

[1] *Department of Psychiatry, Mental Health and Behavioral Sciences, Creighton University*

[2] *Department VA Nebraska- Western Iowa Health Care System 4101 Woolworth Ave Omaha, NE 68105, USA*

[3] *Departments of Psychiatry and Pediatrics, Division of Child and Adolescent Psychiatry, Creighton University, 3528 Dodge Omaha, NE 68131, USA*

[4] *Child and Adolescent Fellowship Training Program, Department of Psychiatry, Creighton University School of Medicine, 3528 Dodge Street Omaha, NE 68131 USA*

[5] *Baptist Health System, 517, Crowne Woods Drive, Birmingham, AL, 35244 USA*

Abstract: Sedative Hypnotic Agents (SHAs) are prescribed across several medical disciplines, however, these carry a risk of addiction in small percentage of patients. SHA use for more than a month can result in tolerance and pharmacological dependence. This often requires dose escalation during the first 10-12 weeks of treatment . This pharmacological dependence should be distinguished from SHA use disorder. In this chapter we discuss the factors associated with risk and risk mitigation for SHA use disorder. Use of lowest possible effective dose for shorter period of time with close monitoring a valuable strategy to prevent addiction. Sudden SHA withdrawal specially from barbiturates may be fatal. We discuss the safe strategy for acute withdrawal by converting the drug of addiction to equivalent dose of a long half-life benzodiazepine or barbiturate. Stabilizing on that drug dose and gradually tapering from that. We also suggest treatment with adjunctive medications for comorbid psychiatric disorders. We conclude this chapter with a brief discussion of psychosocial strategies to promote abstinence and recovery.

* **Corresponding author Subhash C. Bhatia:** Department of Psychiatry, Mental Health and Behavioral Sciences, Creighton University; Department VA Nebraska- Western Iowa Health Care System 4101 Woolworth Ave Omaha, NE 68105, USA; Tel/Fax: (402) 995-4315/(402)995-4240; Email: sub55@cox.net

Subhash C. Bhatia (Ed.)

Keywords: Barbiturates, Benzodiazepines, Benzodiazepine daily equivalents, Dependence, Pharmacological dependence, Sedative Hypnotic use disorders, Withdrawal.

KEY LEARNING POINTS

1. Sedative, hypnotic or anxiolytic (SHA) medications at therapeutic doses are safe and effective in the management of anxiety and insomnia. They have anticonvulsant and muscle relaxant properties. Intoxication results in symptoms like slurred speech, lack of coordination, unsteady gait, and impaired performance while operating machinery or motor vehicles.
2. Chronic use of sedatives, hypnotics and anxiolytics cause pharmacological dependence. Sudden cessation or a significant reduction in dose can cause withdrawal symptoms like tachycardia, tremor, insomnia, anxiety, and agitation. Transient hallucinations and grand mal seizures can occur during severe withdrawal.
3. "Z-drugs" like eszopiclone, zaleplon and zolpidem, zolpidem-ER are nonbezodiazepine sedative hypnotics. These are safe and effective with intermittent and short-term use.
4. Barbiturates and related agents are prescribed infrequently. They cause more euphoria than benzodiazepines; thereby have a higher risk of abuse. Both barbiturate overdose and withdrawal is more dangerous than with other sedative medications.

CLINICAL VIGNETTE

A 27 year-old college student was diagnosed with panic disorder by her primary care physician and was treated with alprazolam 0.5mg three times a day. The dose was gradually increased to 2 mg three times a day over 2 months period. The patient was given monthly prescriptions, but she would call for bridge prescriptions between appointments, citing reasons like losing her prescription medication or accidentally flushing the medication. Her primary care provider assertively communicated to her about misuse of alprazolam, diagnosed her having alprazolam use disorder, and requested a psychiatric consultation.

Psychiatric history revealed that she has been suffering from panic attacks since her teenage years. She had been coping with this anxiety with consumption of heavy amounts of alcohol that provided a temporary relief. She reported that she has been abstinent from alcohol for over a year. She also reported previous cannabis and methamphetamine use, but they made her anxiety and panic symptoms worse and therefore quit using those. Though she initially used alprazolam as prescribed, during her third visit she disclosed consuming at least 10-12 mg of alprazolam a day during the previous 6 months. She reported that dose reduction caused an exacerbation of anxiety symptoms, hand tremors and insomnia. She confided that she was obtaining alprazolam prescription from two different providers, using two different pharmacies. She shared her constant fear about running out of alprazolam. She reported that she felt tired during the day. Her supervisor reprimanded her for missing work, for poor work performance and for frequent work related errors.

For panic disorder, sertraline 25 mg/day was started that was increased to 50 mg/day in a week. The alprazolam dose of 12 mg a day was converted to equivalent benzodiazepine dose of clonazepam 6 mg a day given as 3 mg twice a day. In addition, she was prescribed alprazolam 0.5 mg as needed daily for breakthrough symptoms. The dose of clonazepam was reduced slowly by 0.5 mg every week to a target dose of 0.5 mg twice a day. Following this initial dose reduction regimen, clonazepam was tapered more gradually at 0.25 mg a week. With this slow taper over 9 weeks period, the patient did not experience any rebound or recurrence of symptoms. Along with the medication changes patient engaged in cognitive behavioral therapy to address both panic disorder and substance use disorder.

DISCUSSION OF THE VIGNETTE

Diagnostic Considerations

The patient in this vignette had a long-standing history of anxiety and panic disorder used alcohol to cope with it use disorder. Alcohol, cannabis and methamphetamine use were probable attempts to seek relief from her anxiety symptoms. Stimulant use or abstinence from alcohol increased anxiety and panic symptoms. Tolerance of high doses of alprazolam, withdrawal symptoms on dose reduction, continuing drug use despite adverse consequences like occupational difficulties and drug seeking behaviors *i.e.* use of two providers and two pharmacies, established the diagnosis of anxiolytic use disorder. These diagnostic elements are consistent with diagnostic criteria described in Diagnostic and Statistical Manual of Mental Disorder Fifth Edition (DSM-5) [1].

DSM-5 [1] describes SHA use disorder as problematic use of these substances leading to clinically significant impairment or distress manifested by at least 2 out of 11 diagnostic criteria within 12 months period. These criteria are: use of large doses of SHAs over longer period; persistent desire or unsuccessful efforts to cut down their use, great deal of time spent to obtain these substances; craving or having strong urge to reuse these substances; recurrent use despite failure to meet major role obligations, continued use despite social or interpersonal problems; reducing or giving up participation with family and social or recreational activities due to use of these substances; placing oneself in hazardous situation following their use for example driving while under the influence; continued use despite having physical or psychological problems; developing tolerance or experiencing withdrawal symptoms with cessation or reduction of amount used. This is considered mild if 2-3 symptoms, moderate if presence of 4-5 symptoms and severe with presence of 6 or more symptoms. If a person is without symptoms for 3 months but less than 12 months it is designated early remission, more than 12 months it is sustained remission. With these designations of early or sustained remission add in a controlled environment for example when person is incarcerated. Past history of anxiety or panic symptoms or use of alcohol or these substances increase risk of developing SHA use disorder. Our patient in this vignette met criteria for SHA use disorder with significant impairment in social occupational or role functions.

Management Considerations

Switching to long acting benzodiazepine like clonazepam and tapering it slowly is a common strategy [2]. Selective Serotonin Reuptake Inhibitors (SSRI) like sertraline [3] and Cognitive Behavioral Therapy (CBT) [4] are well-recognized interventions for panic disorder. Treating anxiety disorder further improves the outcomes of substance use disorder.

Diagnosis of sedative, hypnotic or anxiolytic (SHA) related disorders are diagnosed through detailed history from the patient and collateral sources, physical and mental status examination, and urine drug screen. SHA's have anti-anxiety, anticonvulsant, muscle relaxant and sedative properties. Benzodiazepines have relatively low abuse potential, as well as a low lethality index following an overdose; this is not the case with barbiturate overdose. In therapeutic doses for known indications benzodiazepines are safe and effective and help improve the quality of life. Four or more weeks of continuous SHA therapy often results in pharmacological dependence. Addiction to SHA's develops in a small minority of patients. This risk is higher in those with a past history of substance use and comorbid psychiatric disorder. These drugs can cause sedation and impairment of motor functions with impairment of ability to operate machinery or drive a motor vehicle safely. In addition, cognitive dysfunction may be caused by benzodiazepines [5] leading to errors executing cognitive tasks.

SEDATIVE, HYPNOTIC OR ANXIOLYTIC-RELATED DISORDERS IN DSM-5

SHA Use Disorders, SHA Intoxication, SHA withdrawal, other SHA-Induced disorders and unspecified SHA-Related Disorder [1].

NEUROPSYCHOPHARMACOLOGY

All SHAs have affinity for gamma-amino butyric acid (GABA) receptors specifically GABA A subtype. Further subtypes of GABA A receptor are alpha, beta, gamma etc. The GABA as an agonist of these receptors opens the chloride channels causing over polarizing the neuron with net result of inhibition of neuron. There are many subunits of alpha subunit. Out of these alpha 1 subunit is associated with hypnotic, anticonvulsant and amnestic effects. Adaption of this subunit leads to tolerance and withdrawal. Benzodiazepine work through agonist effect on alpha 1, 2, and 3 subunits. Effect of alpha 2 and 3 subunits results in anxiolytic effects. "Z" drugs work through agonism of alpha 1 subunit there by sedation and no anxiolytic effect. Chronic use leads to tolerance due to adaptation of these receptors and sudden stoppage to withdrawal. Slow and gradual taper decreases risk of serious withdrawal.

EPIDEMIOLOGY

The medical use of sedative, hypnotic and anxiolytics has decreased in general. The prescription utilization of these drugs is more common in whites, women and elderly population. The National Institute on Drug Abuse's National Household Survey 2011 reports that 22.5 million Americans 12 years or older reported use of illicit drug during the month prior to the survey interview. In this survey, 0.1% report sedative use and 0.7% report tranquilizers use. The mean age of first illicit use of sedatives is 22 years and 24.6 years for tranquilizers [7].

PHARMACOLOGICAL DEPENDENCE *VS.* ADDICTION

Benzodiazepine use for more than a month can cause pharmacological dependence. The tolerance to sedation is usually greater than the anxiolytic effects. Often patients require 2-3 increments in dosage in the first 10-12 weeks following benzodiazepine initiation. The pharmacological dependence requiring dose increment should not be confused with addiction. However pharmacological dependence is associated with a risk of developing discontinuation/withdrawal syndrome, characterized by autonomic hyperactivity, hand tremor, agitation, anxiety, grand mal seizures, rebound or recurrence of anxiety symptoms. Risk of withdrawal is higher with high potency, high doses, and shorter acting benzodiazepines with abrupt discontinuation. As opposed to pharmacological dependence, addiction refers to illicit and nonmedical use of these drugs, craving to reuse, with drug seeking behavior as well as compulsive use despite adverse social, occupational, cognitive, affective and behavioral consequences.

Barbiturates through their greater effect on the reward circuits also add to addictive potential. Short and intermediate half-life barbiturates like amobarbital, pentobarbital and secobarbital have a limited clinical role due to narrow therapeutic index and a higher risk of fatal outcome in overdose. Chloral hydrate for sleep and phenobarbital for seizure disorders continued to be used.

FACTORS THAT MAY CONTRIBUTE TO SEDATIVE, HYPNOTIC OR ANXIOLYTIC USE DISORDER

Patient Related Factors

History of sedative abuse, alcohol abuse and dependence; family history of drug abuse or dependence; chronic anxiety and panic disorder; unrecognized comorbid depression, personality factors like poor coping and poor interpersonal skills, and limited social support system increases the risk of SHA use disorder.

Drug Pharmacokinetic or Pharmacodynamics Related Factors

Rapid onset of action, high lipid solubility with rapid crossing of the blood brain barrier and experience of a drug related "buzz" or "high". This high may be reinforcing and conducive to reuse or misuse. Prolonged use of high dose and high potency SHA's with a short half life can lead to inter dose rebound anxiety or panic symptoms and may also promote reuse of drug.

Drug Availability Related Factor

Prescription of high doses in patients with benzodiazepine non-responsive conditions and frequent use of high potency short half-life medication on an as required basis (PRN) promotes clock-watching behavior. When the paradigm of symptom, medication, relief, and reinforcement operates multiple times a day every day PRN dosing is likely to increase the risk of psychological dependence. Also prescribing inadequate doses may increase the risk of dependence, as patient may self-escalate the dose for symptom relief. This pattern is also conducive to drug dependence. Easy access to these drugs for nonmedical use often contributes to use disorder.

Sedative, Hypnotic or Anxiolytic Use Disorders: Risk Reduction

To optimize therapeutic use and reduce the risk of SHA addiction, consider using only in disorders responsive to these drugs, using the lowest required dose, for the shortest possible time and after weighing the risk and benefits. These medication prescriptions should be monitored closely. Prescription should be based on scheduled dosing, and as needed therapy especially short half-life drugs should be avoided. Consider non-benzodiazepine non habit forming pharmacologic alternatives for generalized anxiety like buspirone, a 5 HT1a agonist, hydroxyzine, serotonin selective reuptake inhibitors for anxiety and panic disorder and non-pharmacologic therapies like cognitive-behavior therapy, coping and social skills training, relaxation therapy, yoga and physical exercise. For sleep if warranted alternative therapy with, antihistamines, trazodone, mirtazapine, doxepin and amitriptyline may be considered. If the decision is to stop the medication, taper it slowly in an individualized manner to prevent rebound symptoms and minimize withdrawal related distress. Urine drug screening helps identify non prescribed drug use, however some benzodiazepines like clonazepam can be missed on routine urine drug screen.

Managing Withdrawal

Detoxification from barbiturates [8] requires converting the total daily dose of barbiturates to an equivalent phenobarbital dose using the conversion factor e.g. 100 mg of amobarbital, butabarbital, butalbital, pentobarbital and secobarbital being equal to 30 mg of phenobarbital. The phenobarbital equivalent dose should be administered in three doses spread across the day. However, before administering each phenobarbital dose the patient should be evaluated for slurred speech, nystagmus and ataxia. Sustained nystagmus is the most reliable sign of intoxication, and when present the scheduled dose of phenobarbital should be held. Experiencing acute withdrawal symptoms following a phenobarbital dose places the patient at a high risk for seizures, and an intramuscular dose of phenobarbital should be administered. Presence of nystagmus within 1-2 hours after phenobarbital injection is indicative of a limited risk of withdrawal. Once the daily phenobarbital equivalent dose is established (See Table **2**), the patient should be stabilized on the dose for 2 days, followed by a gradual dose reduction of usually 30 mg per day or a slower taper if withdrawal symptoms manifest.

Withdrawal symptoms peak between 5 to 10 days and rarely can last up to a year. Withdrawal should be accomplished with an individualized gradual benzodiazepine dose reduction. With short-term use, the first half of the drug may be tapered at a rate of 25% every 3-5 days (we used a slower strategy in our patient), and the second half of the dose should be reduced more slowly. One of the common strategies in tapering these medications is to convert the drug from a short acting to mg equivalent dose of a long acting benzodiazepine using the conversion factors in Table **1**. For the patient in our vignette we converted 12 mg alprazolam to 6 mg of clonazepam [2]. For breakthrough symptoms, we allowed 0.5 mg of alprazolam on as needed basis to minimize distress from withdrawal symptoms. However with more chronic use, 50% of the medication can be reduced in 4 weeks and the other half is weaned off over few months. With high potency medications like clonazepam and alprazolam, slower taper at 0.5mg every 2-3 weeks is necessary to prevent withdrawal symptoms. When in doubt, daily benzodiazepine use can be estimated by administering the patient 1mg clonazepam every 1-2 hours until the patient is free of withdrawal symptoms. Once the 24-hour requirement is known, the same dose should be administered on twice a day dosing, with a planned gradual reduction by 10% every week. Withdrawal from zolpidem and zopiclone is not common to the extent rebound insomnia is rare in clinical trials; however withdrawal delirium and seizures have been reported with high doses. The withdrawal symptoms can be addressed with a downward titration of the same drug or using a long acting benzodiazepine like diazepam.

Table 1. Benzodiazepine equivalence and half-life.

	Equivalent Dose to 5 mg Diazepam	**Half-Life of Drug**
Alprazolam	0.5 mg	Short
Chlordiazepoxide	10 mg	Long
Clonazepam	0.25 mg	Long
Clorazepate	7.5 mg	Long
Flurazepam	15 mg	Long
Lorazepam	1 mg	Short
Oxazepam	15 mg	Short
Temazepam	15 mg	Short
Triazolam	0.125 mg	Very short

Adapted from references [12, 13]

Table 2. Barbiturate and related drugs equivalence table.

	Equivalent to 30 mg Phenobarbital	Half-life
Amobarbital	100 mg	Intermediate
Butabarbital	100 mg	Intermediate
Butalbital	100 mg	Intermediate
Pentobarbital	100 mg	Short
Secobarbital	100 mg	Intermediate
Chloral hydrate	500 mg	Long

Adapted from reference [12]

PROMOTING RECOVERY

Pharmacological Interventions

Along with managing withdrawal, it is important to promote abstinence. A Cochrane review found tapering the benzodiazepine dose over 10 weeks to reduce dropout rates and did not find the switch to long acting benzodiazepines useful [9]. Valproate, lamotrigine and carbamazepine have GABA agonist properties, providing an additional advantage of prophylaxis against withdrawal seizures. These can be used for gradual discontinuation of benzodiazepines and maintain abstinence [10]. Infusing flumazenil during benzodiazepine withdrawal is a novel approach showing promise in reducing withdrawal symptoms and improving abstinence [11]. Comorbid substance use and psychiatric conditions are common with SHA use their treatment improves prognosis.

Psychological Interventions

Motivational enhancement and cognitive behavioral therapy (CBT) approaches are effective. CBT addresses cognitive distortions around benefits of the sedatives, withdrawal and coping without sedatives.

Social Interventions

Narcotics Anonymous a spirituality-based 12-step program and peer support from a ‘sponsor’ can be valuable in promoting recovery.

SUMMARY

SHAs when used under clinical supervision are safe and effective, alleviate debilitating anxiety and insomnia and thereby improve the quality of life. However, a minority of individuals develop addiction. The risk is higher in those with limited social and coping skills, a family or past history of substance use disorder, comorbid psychiatric disorders and in those who are seeking a medication induced "high". This patient population is likely to develop drug dependence requiring drug rehabilitation.

BENZODIAZEPINES - PATIENT EDUCATION HANDOUT

What are Benzodiazepines?

These medications are from the diazepam (Valium) family. They are prescribed for anxiety related conditions, seizures and sleep problems.

What are Anxiety Related Conditions?

These are conditions where patient experiences psychological symptoms like excessive worry, feeling tense, and have physical symptoms like palpitations, shortness of breath, butterflies in the stomach and tremors (shakes). Some times patients actively avoid triggers for the anxiety.

Will I Get Addicted to Benzodiazepines?

Benzodiazepine addiction is rare but can happen. A family history of addictions, poor coping and social skills, high dose self-directed benzodiazepine use, and other addictions increase the risk of benzodiazepine addiction.

What will Happen if I Chose to Stop My Benzodiazepines Suddenly?

If you are taking a benzodiazepine for 30 days or longer, then stopping it suddenly can result in withdrawal symptoms. These symptoms could range from symptoms of anxiety, confusion, hallucinations and even seizures.

What is the Role of Barbiturates in the Treatment of Sleep Disorders?

Barbiturates except phenobarbital are prescribed rarely. These drugs have a greater tendency for habit forming and are more dangerous than benzodiazepines both in overdose and abrupt discontinuation.

Barbiturates are Prescribed Rarely. How does Barbiturate Addiction Occur?

Patients with barbiturate addiction often buy these drugs from the streets. Using frequent and high dosages of these drugs cause addiction.

What Sleeping Medications I Should Ask for So that I do not Get Addicted?

New sleeping medications like Ambien, Ambien-CR, Lunesta, and Sonata are "Z-drugs". They are safe and effective when used intermittently for a shorter period. These medications should be taken just before going to sleep. Please note that your body might get used to these medications and abrupt discontinuation can cause a return of sleep problems.

What is the Use of Talk Therapy to Come Off Benzodiazepines?

During benzodiazepine reduction, anxiety may return or rebound. Talk therapy (psychotherapy) helps to understand what is expected during withdrawal, promotes coping skills and confidence in coming off and staying off these drugs.

What are the Other Treatment Options for My Anxiety?

Medications like buspirone and certain antidepressants like Zoloft (sertraline), and talk therapies like cognitive behavioral therapy are used to treat anxiety disorders.

CONFLICT OF INTEREST

The authors confirm that they have no conflict of interest to declare for this publication.

ACKNOWLEDGEMENTS

Declared none.

REFERENCES

[1] Diagnostic and Statistical Manual of Mental Disorders. 5th ed., Arlington, VA: American Psychiatric Association 2013.

[2] Herman JB, Rosenbaum JF, Brotman AW. The alprazolam to clonazepam switch for the treatment of panic disorder. J Clin Psychopharmacol 1987; 7(3): 175-8.
[http://dx.doi.org/10.1097/00004714-198706000-00012] [PMID: 3597803]

[3] Pohl RB, Wolkow RM, Clary CM. Sertraline in the treatment of panic disorder: a double-blind multicenter trial. Am J Psychiatry 1998; 155(9): 1189-95.
[http://dx.doi.org/10.1176/ajp.155.9.1189] [PMID: 9734541]

[4] Otto MW, Deveney C. Cognitive-behavioral therapy and the treatment of panic disorder: efficacy and strategies. J Clin Psychiatry 2005; 66 (Suppl. 4): 28-32.
[PMID: 15842185]

[5] Barker MJ, Greenwood KM, Jackson M, Crowe SF. Cognitive effects of long-term benzodiazepine use: a meta-analysis. CNS Drugs 2004; 18(1): 37-48.
[http://dx.doi.org/10.2165/00023210-200418010-00004] [PMID: 14731058]

[6] Stahl SM. Stahl's essential psychopharmacology: neuroscientific basis and practical application. 4th ed., Cambridge, United Kingdom: Cambridge University Press 2013.

[7] Results from the 2011 National Survey on Drug Use and Health: Summary of National Findings, NSDUH Series H-44, HHS Publication No (SMA) 12-4713. Rockville, MD: Substance Abuse and Mental Health Services Administration 2012.

[8] Smith DE, Wesson DR. A phenobarbital technique for withdrawal of barbiturate abuse. Arch Gen Psychiatry 1971; 24: 56-60.
[http://dx.doi.org/10.1001/archpsyc.1971.01750070058007] [PMID: 5538852]

[9] Denis C, Fatséas M, Lavie E, Auriacombe M. Pharmacological interventions for benzodiazepine mono-dependence management in outpatient settings. Cochrane Database Syst Rev 2006; (3): CD005194.
[http://dx.doi.org/10.1002/14651858.CD005194.pub2] [PMID: 16856084]

[10] Bisaga A. Benzodiazepines and other sedatives and hypnotics. In: Textbook of substance abuse treatment. 4th ed., Arlington: American Psychiatric Publishing 2008.

[11] Hood S, O'Neil G, Hulse G. The role of flumazenil in the treatment of benzodiazepine dependence: physiological and psychological profiles. J Psychopharmacol (Oxford) 2009; 23(4): 401-9.
[http://dx.doi.org/10.1177/0269881108100322] [PMID: 19164495]

[12] Gautam S, Jain S, Batra L, Lodha P. Clinical practice guidelines for management Of barbiturates and benzodiazepine dependence. Indian J Psychiatry 2006; 66-83.

[13] Shader RI, Greenblatt DJ. Can you provide a table of equivalences for benzodiazepines and other marketed benzodiazepine receptor agonists? J Clin Psychopharmacol 1997; 17(4): 331.
[http://dx.doi.org/10.1097/00004714-199708000-00024] [PMID: 9241022]

CHAPTER 17

Stimulant Use and Addictive Disorder: Amphetamine, Cocaine and Other Stimulants

Prasad R. Padala[1,*] and **Subhash C. Bhatia**[2]

[1] *Clinical, VISN 16 Geriatric Research Education and Clinical Center (GRECC), Deaprtment of Psychiatry and Geriatrics, UAMS, 2200 Fort Roots Drive, North Little Rock, AR 72114, USA*

[2] *Department of Psychiatry, Mental Health and Behavioral Sciences, Creighton University; Department VA Nebraska- Western Iowa Health Care System 4101 Woolworth Ave Omaha, NE 68105, USA*

Abstract: Stimulant and cocaine use disorders are major public health problems. The prevalence of these disorders is on the rise around the globe and within in the US. Often more than one stimulant is used concurrently more often in patients with other psychiatric disorders like depression. These drugs are ingested, injected, smoked or snorted. Short-term effects lasts for about 40-60 minutes for cocaine and up to 12 hours for meth amphetamine, is characterized by initial "rush", increased energy, a general sense of wellbeing, euphoria, increased sex drive, increased self-confidence and decreased appetite, which typically lasts 40-60 minutes for cocaine and 6–12 hours for methamphetamine. Long-term use may result in psychosis and cognitive impairment. The economic, medical and societal impact of these disorders is substantial. The cost increases are due to 24 fold increase in myocardial infarction or infectious diseases like HIV and hepatitis in IV drug users, increased prevalence of psychosis and mood disorders as well as cost incurred by criminal justice system. Cognitive behavioral therapy has been extensively used for stimulant use disorders. Medication management with stimulants and anticonvulsants has shown modest improvement for relapse prevention. Contingency contracting coupled with medication management has resulted in improvement.

* **Corresponding author Prasad R. Padala:** Clinical, VISN 16 Geriatric Research Education and Clinical Center (GRECC), Associate Professor of Psychiatry and Geriatrics, UAMS, 2200 Fort Roots Drive, North Little Rock, AR 72114 USA; Tel: 501-257-2537; Fax; (501) 257-2501; Email: prasad.padala@va.gov

Subhash C. Bhatia (Ed.)

Keywords: Bupropion, Cocaine, "Crack", "Crank", Disulfiram, "Freebase", "Meth", Modafinil, "Speed", Stimulants, Topiramate.

KEY LEARNING POINTS

1. Cocaine, amphetamines and other stimulant use is increasing worldwide with about 43 million people using either cocaine or stimulants.
2. Cocaine and stimulants are consumed in a variety of ways. Powdered form such as "speed," "meth," or "crank" can be snorted, injected, or dissolved in beverages. Freebase methamphetamine is smoked in a pipe or on aluminum foil. Cocaine is used as powder for intranasal or intravenous use, or smoked as crack.
3. It is not uncommon to find that more than one stimulant is used concurrently.
4. Stimulant related disorders are more common in patients with other psychiatric conditions such as depression.
5. Stimulant related disorders are: Stimulant Use Disorder, Stimulant Intoxication, Stimulant Withdrawal and Stimulant-Induced Disorder like Psychosis.
6. Myocardial infarction (MI) is a serious complication of cocaine use.
7. Treatment considerations include cognitive behavioral therapy, contingency management strategies and medications for detoxification and relapse prevention.

CLINICAL VIGNETTE

47 year old single African American male, presented to the Mental Health Clinic with history of relapse of cocaine use. He started to use cocaine at age of 14 years. He stated that he needed more cocaine to get the same "high". He spent a lot of time to procure and use cocaine, had traded sex to obtain cocaine and continued to use it despite knowing its harmful effects. His recent use started after being sober for two months. He used $6000 worth of cocaine in the past two months with the most recent use being three days prior to this visit. He stated he lost about 20 lbs. weight, and had experienced multiple episodes of chest pain during the course of the current relapse. He has not had an EKG recently. His longest sobriety from cocaine use was about four years ago which lasted for about 7 months. Even during early phase of cocaine remission, patient reported to have had an urge to use. Although guarded about history of using other stimulants, he revealed that he

also used methamphetamine about 9 years ago. At that time amount of methamphetamine use was contingent on availability of funds. Based on frequency, amount and duration of use and other behaviors at that time he met the diagnostic criteria for methamphetamine use disorder.

On this visit the patient reported depressed mood and poor concentration. He also reported hearing voices and was distressed because these voices were derogatory and occasionally commenting on his actions. He stated he wants treatment as he was "tired of drug use" and was frustrated with his inability to stop it. He also reported being afraid of medical consequences, particularly because of recent episodes of chest pain and weight loss.

His past psychiatric history was positive for major depressive disorder, recurrent type. He was being treated with bupropion and reported still having residual symptoms of depression. He had history of suicidal thoughts and attempts in the past. His last attempt was about 9 years ago. He has had psychotic symptoms even while not using stimulant(s) actively. He gave a history of physical, emotional and sexual trauma at age 8. He reported nightmares off and on related to his sexual trauma but denied having any flashbacks. He denied any OCD symptoms. His past medical history was positive for hepatitis C, human immunodeficiency virus, hypothyroidism and gastro esophageal reflux disease.

He was born and raised in California and supported himself financially with monthly social security disability check. He admitted to diverting his disability benefits for drug purchases. He was living in public housing by himself and was recently served an eviction notice due to nonpayment of rent. He had never married and did not have any children.

DISCUSSION OF THE VIGNETTE

Recognition

In this vignette, the patient presented three days after the last use of cocaine and did not have any short-term effects. He met the diagnostic criteria for stimulant use disorder and major depression. Generally short-term effects of stimulant use present as initial "rush", increased energy, a general sense of wellbeing, euphoria, increased sex drive, increased self-confidence and decreased appetite, which typically lasts 40-60 minutes for cocaine and 6-12 hours for methamphetamine. Also often patients have increased blood pressure, body temperature, heart rate, cardiac arrhythmias and increased breathing rate, motor restlessness, insomnia, hyperthermia, bruxism, and possibly convulsions.

Long-term use can lead to addiction, paranoia, mood disturbances, agitation, psychosis, and cognitive impairment. The patient in this vignette presented with depression and psychosis perhaps as long-term deleterious effects of stimulant use. Methamphetamine-induced psychosis can be long lasting and may even present in the absence of further drug use. The patient presented did have psychotic symptoms even when not using stimulants. Violence due to delusions is not uncommon. Amphetamine use can also result in delirium manifested by disorientation, confusion, fear, and anxiety. Following prolonged use, discontinuation of stimulants often results in a withdrawal syndrome including dysphoric mood, fatigue, sleep disturbances, psychomotor agitation or retardation, vivid and unpleasant dreams and increased appetite. Methamphetamine withdrawal symptoms last longer than those associated with cocaine. Cue-induced cravings in the late stages of withdrawal are common like driving by "crack house" and start to experience craving.

Diagnostic Considerations

A clear history from patient and collateral sources, mental status examination augmented with drug screens are important for diagnose of stimulant use disorder. Use of more than one drug in conjunction with alcohol is more a rule than exception, many patients with cocaine dependence also use methamphetamine as was the case in our patient. 60-80% of cocaine dependent patients are also alcohol dependent [1]. Euphoria associated with cocaine or methamphetamine intoxication is hard to distinguish from a manic episode. Collaborative history about drug use from friends or family members is important to make the distinction. A high degree of suspicion is essential particularly in settings such as emergency rooms. Dysphoria associated with the withdrawal from these agents can be mistakenly diagnosed as major depressive disorder. Methamphetamine psychosis can be confused with schizophrenia although the predominance of visual and tactile hallucinations may give a clue about drug related etiology. Drug screen can be helpful in making the distinction although in many cases psychosis induced by chronic methamphetamine use may persist long after stopping the use of the drug.

An increased rate of serious mental illness is found which in turn increases the risk of substance use. Patients with schizophrenia are known to use stimulants to decrease the negative symptoms. Risk of HIV infection is increased particularly with intravenous methamphetamine use and/or unprotected sex. Hepatitis C is also common.

Special considerations in geriatric population: Contrary to traditional wisdom, recent literature has shown that substance use may not stop with aging. With the tide of baby boomers reaching the geriatric age, illicit drug use is a huge concern. The National Household Survey on Drug Abuse (NHSDA) found that among adults between 50-59 years, the rate of current illicit drug use increased from 1.9% in 2002 to 4.1% in 2007 [2]. Drug use may even start late in life. In a study of 117 veterans aged 50 and older treated for crack cocaine, 14.5% began their cocaine abuse after the age of 50 [3]. In a suburban community hospital in over 10,000 drug screens, 22.7% tested positive for cocaine, including 2.3% in those aged 65 and older [4]. Cocaine abuse is seen in older adults and often goes undiagnosed. Reluctance of physicians and health care providers to ask about drug use in elderly could contribute to underdiagnosis. A high degree of suspicion and regular screening may improve the identification of cocaine and stimulant abuse. Cardiovascular effects of stimulants and cocaine are of particular concern in elderly. Special attention needs to be paid to the social consequences and caregiver burden associated with stimulant use in older adults.

Cocaine and Stimulant Related Disorders

In DSM-5 [5] these are classified as, Stimulant use disorder, Stimulant Intoxication, Stimulant Withdrawal, Other or unspecified Stimulant use disorders. The diagnostic criteria for all of these categories are described in detail in DSM-5.

EPIDEMIOLOGY

Stimulant and cocaine related disorders are major public health problems because of their psychological, social and medical impacts, including the impact on fetus with use during pregnancy and spread of infectious diseases such as HIV, hepatitis B and C and tuberculosis. Stimulants can generally be categorized into cocaine and amphetamine-like substances as they have similar clinical presentation, outcome and complications. Amphetamine-type substances come in several different forms and can be administered in many routes. Powdered form such as "speed", "meth", or "crank" can be snorted, injected, or dissolved in beverages. Freebase methamphetamine can also be smoked in a pipe or on aluminum foil [6]. Cocaine is used as powder for intranasal or intravenous use, or smoked as crack. Medical prescriptions of dexamphetamine, methylphenidate or illegally manufactured methamphetamine powder are commonly preferred by patients with stimulant use disorder.

Prevalence of stimulant use disorders is on the rise worldwide. Cocaine use is highly prevalent and remains under-treated. In 2007 in the US alone there were 2.5 million individuals with cocaine dependence, of whom only 809,000 received treatment [7]. Cocaine use has remained at the same levels in the past five years [8]. 30 million people worldwide use amphetamine-type stimulants, primarily methamphetamine, compared with an estimated 13 million who use cocaine [9]. In the US methamphetamine is the preferred amphetamine and its abuse has increased substantially. Stimulant use disproportionately increases the health care costs associated with several complications of their use. Cocaine dependence alone accounts for a third of drug-related emergency department visits in the US and has substantial social and economic burden [10].

MEDICAL ISSUES WITH COCAINE AND STIMULANTS

Myocardial infarction (MI) is a serious complication of cocaine use. These patients typically present to the emergency room with chest pain after a recent ingestion of cocaine irrespective of the route of intake. Hence it is prudent to inquire about cocaine use while working up chest pain in the ER. In those that use cocaine, the risk of acute MI is increased as much as 24 times compared to healthy individuals [11]. Cocaine is a potent coronary vasoconstrictor due to its actions on the sympathetic nervous system. In addition to the coronary vasoconstriction, it also contributes to increased myocardial oxygen consumption and thrombus formation. Hypertension and cardiac arrhythmias are other cardiovascular complications of cocaine use. Its use has also been linked to seizures, hyperpyrexia, rhabdomyalisis, and perforation of the nasal septum [12]. Strokes and massive intracerebral hemorrhages have been reported with methamphetamine use. Methamphetamine use has also been linked to higher risk of HIV due to increased sexual drive and disinhibition during methamphetamine intoxication. Poor dentition or so called "meth mouth" is frequently present.

TREATMENT CONSIDERATIONS

Pharmacological Interventions

There are no FDA approved medications for stimulant use disorders.

Non-FDA approved pharmacotherapy for stimulant dependence can be broadly classified into medicines used for detoxification and those used for relapse prevention.

Detoxification Pharmacotherapy

Drugs with psychostimulant properties are useful as substitution agents. Drugs such as methylphenidate, modafinil, bupropion, and selegeline have been used for detoxification from cocaine use. A Cochrane review concluded that these agents did not improve overall cocaine use, had an unclear beneficial effect over sustained cocaine abstinence and were not associated with higher retention in treatment [13]. However, they were beneficial for some groups of patients, such as methadone maintained dual heroin-cocaine addicts. A recent review on this topic revealed the strongest evidence for substitution therapies for amphetamine analogs or dopaminergic agents combined with contingency management [14].

Grabowski and associates found that higher dose of dextroamphetamine (30-60 mg per day) was superior to both lower dose (15-30 mg per day) and placebo for treatment of cocaine dependence [15]. Modafinil is FDA approved for excessive day time sleepiness associated with narcolepsy. It has been used for detoxification in patients with cocaine dependence and also abstinence by blocking the euphoric effects of cocaine [16, 17]. In a large, multicenter, randomized controlled trial modafinil reduced cocaine cravings and increased cocaine non-use days in subjects without comorbid alcohol dependence [17]. Modafinil may be effective due to its mild stimulant properties that might help in reducing the withdrawal from cocaine and also its glutamate enhancing properties. One concern with modafinil is insomnia as it promotes wakefulness however a recent report suggests that modafinil reversed polysomnographic abnormalities in twenty cocaine-dependent patients during supervised abstinence [18].

Bupropion has been tried in stimulant dependence due to its dopamine and norepinephrine reuptake inhibitor properties. Mixed results have been reported in its usefulness in stimulant dependence. Although randomized controlled trials failed to separate bupropion from placebo in either cocaine and metham-phematimine dependence, concurrent use of contingency management with bupropion may result in significant improvement in outcomes in cocaine addiction [19 - 21]. In another study levodopa combined with vouchers, a contingency management strategy, was associated with higher rates of abstinence and higher proportions of cocaine-free urines [22].

Relapse Prevention Pharmacotherapy

Since cocaine increases dopamine in the mesocortical areas of the brain, GABergic and glutaminergic agents have been used in relapse prevention as these agents have inhibitory effect on the dopaminergic neurotransmission. Vigabatrin is a novel antiepileptic that irreversibly inhibits GABA-transaminase. Two small open label studies have shown promising results with vigabatrin in maintaining abstinence from cocaine use [23, 24]. In a recent randomized controlled trial with the same agent, full end-of-trial abstinence was achieved in 28.0% of the vigabatrin treated subjects *versus* 7.5% of those in the placebo arm. Additionally vigabatrin use was associated with superior self-reported full end-of-trial abstinence from alcohol (43.5% *versus* 6.3%) [25]. Visual field defects have been associated with long-term use of vigabatrin although these defects were not seen with short trials of vigabatrin.

Topiramate, another antiepileptic with dual actions on GABA-ergic and glutaminergic neurotransmission, has been used successfully in reducing cravings for cocaine, and abstinence from cocaine use [26, 27]. A combination of topiramate with mixed amphetamine salts was found to be more effective in promoting cocaine abstinence in patients with severe cocaine dependence [28]. Topiramate was also found to be effective in reducing relapse rates in methamphetamine dependence [29].

Pre-treatment with disulfiram increases cocaine and dopamine levels after cocaine intake leading to high levels of anxiety and thus helps in abstinence. A recent Cochrane review found a trend favoring disulfiram on number of weeks of abstinence from cocaine compared to placebo [30].

Promising results are seen with a cocaine vaccine given in five intramuscular injections substantially decreased smoked cocaine's intoxicating effects in those generating sufficient antibody [31]. In a double-blind placebo controlled trial in methadone controlled subjects significant reduction in cocaine use was seen in those that developed high IgG anticocaine antibodies [32]. Studies are ongoing to increase the antibody response to the vaccine.

Adrenergic blockers have been used to treat stimulant dependence. Propranolol reduces anxiety during withdrawal and may also blunt cocaine-induced euphoria and craving [33].

Drugs under development: Lofexidine, an α2-adrenergic agonist, reduces the craving induced by stress and drug cues in drug users, suggesting utility as a treatment for stimulant addiction. In addition, the norepinephrine transporter (NET) inhibitor atomoxetine attenuates some of d-amphetamine's subjective and physiological effects. Cocaine dependence is linked with white matter impairments. A recent study [34] used diffusion tensor imaging (DTI), a novel radiologic technique to measure white matter integrity, in 16 patients with cocaine dependence. They found a positive correlation of cocaine abstinence and cocaine free urine drug tests with white matter integrity. Authors suggest that future treatments of cocaine dependence also focus on improving the white matter integrity.

Psychological Interventions

The typical syndrome associated with stimulant intoxication is acute agitation, which may often best be handled by talking down the patient, assuring them that the condition will pass in time, while observing them and ensuring a calm environment. If recent stimulant administration indicates the possibility of toxicity, measures may be taken to promote clearance of the drug; emetics or lavage may be useful in removing amphetamine pills, but much more common is toxicity from intravenous or smoked stimulants. Currently, there are no medications that can quickly and safely reverse a life-threatening stimulant overdose. In severe cases, when potential for harm to self or others is manifest, either a benzodiazepine or an antipsychotic may be used. Clinicians should observe for and treat possible dehydration and hyperthermia.

Individual, group and family therapy has been effective treatment for stimulant dependence. Cognitive behavioral therapy has been extensively used. Contingency contracting has been used with stimulant dependence with some success.

Social Interventions

Cocaine Anonymous (CA) patterned after Alcoholic Anonymous with a sponsor has proven beneficial for some patients. Appointment of a payee to manage funds can reduce diversion of funds for drug purchases.

SUMMARY

Stimulant and cocaine use disorders are major public health problems. Unfortunately the prevalence of stimulant dependence is on the rise worldwide and within in the US. The economic, medical and societal impact of stimulant use disorders is substantial. It is not uncommon to find that more than one stimulant is used concurrently. Stimulant related disorders are more common in patients with other psychiatric conditions such as depression. Numerous medical complications result with stimulant use disorders increasing the cost of caring for such patients. The risk of myocardial infarction is increased 24 fold in patients with cocaine use disorder compared to those without. Cognitive behavioral therapy has been extensively used for stimulant use disorders. Medication management has shown modest improvement with stimulant like medications and anticonvulsants for relapse prevention. Contingency contracting coupled with medication management has resulted in relapse prevention.

STIMULANT RELATED DISORDERS - PATIENT EDUCATION SHEET

What is a Stimulant?

Stimulants are a group of medications which when ingested stimulate the central nervous system. These drugs include cocaine and amphetamine-like substances. Amphetamine-type substances include powder like substance commonly known as “speed,” “meth,” or “crank”. These powder like substances are often snorted, injected, or dissolved in beverages. Freebase methamphetamine is also smoked in a pipe or on aluminum foil. Cocaine is available as white powder that is either used intranasally or injected, or smoked as crack. Medical prescriptions of dexamphetamine, methylphenidate or illegally manufactured methamphetamine powder are also abused as stimulants.

What are Symptoms of Stimulant Intoxication?

Symptoms of stimulant intoxication include a sense of euphoria, heightened sense of well-being, increased energy, agitation, restlessness, irritability, rapid shifts in thinking, hypervigilence, poor concentration and poor impulse control. Patients with stimulant intoxication often present with increased heart rate, blood pressure, profuse sweating, suppressed appetite, insomnia and teeth grinding.

What are the Withdrawal Effects of Stimulants Use?

Withdrawal symptoms develop hours to days after heavy use stops. Patients present with dysphoria or frank depression. Depression can be severe in those with pre-existing depression. They also present with loss of interest in pleasurable activities, social withdrawal, anxiety, impaired memory and intense cravings. They often present with fatigue, dehydration, hunger, dulled senses and insomnia.

Are Stimulants Addictive?

Yes. Some people are at higher risk of addiction than others. A family history of depression or other mental illness, past history of mental illness, use of other drugs can put someone at higher risk of developing addiction to stimulants.

What Medical Complications can be Caused by Stimulants?

Numerous medical complications result with stimulant use disorders. The risk of myocardial infarction is increased 24 fold in patients with cocaine use disorder compared to those without. High blood pressure and rhythm abnormalities of the heart are also complications of cocaine use. Its use has also been linked to seizures, and perforation of the nasal septum. Strokes and bleeding in the brain have been reported with methamphetamine use. Methamphetamine use has also been linked to higher risk of HIV due to increased sexual drive and disinhibition during methamphetamine intoxication.

How is Stimulant Related Disorder Diagnosed?

Stimulant related disorders are diagnosed clinically by obtaining detailed history from patient and collateral sources, conducting physical and mental status evaluation and utilizing current diagnostic criteria. Laboratory investigations can further strengthen the diagnosis.

How are Stimulant Use Disorders Treated?

Psychotherapy has been the mainstay of treatment with cognitive behavioral therapy as the most studied modality. Medications are used to detoxify and also prevent relapse. Combination of medications with contingency planning may have added benefits. It is important to treat other co-occurring conditions such as depression and medical complications.

CONFLICT OF INTEREST

The authors confirm that they have no conflict of interest to declare for this publication.

ACKNOWLEDGEMENTS

Declared none.

REFERENCES

[1] Carroll KM, Rounsaville BJ, Bryant KJ. Alcoholism in treatment-seeking cocaine abusers: clinical and prognostic significance. J Stud Alcohol 1993; 54(2): 199-208. [http://dx.doi.org/10.15288/jsa.1993.54.199] [PMID: 8459714]

[2] Gfroerer J, Penne M, Pemberton M, Folsom R. Substance abuse treatment need among older adults in 2020: the impact of the aging baby-boom cohort. Drug Alcohol Depend 2003; 69(2): 127-35. [http://dx.doi.org/10.1016/S0376-8716(02)00307-1] [PMID: 12609694]

[3] Dianna T, James B. American Association for Geriatric Psychiatry 21st Annual Meeting Poster 60; 2004.

[4] Chait R, Fahmy S, Caceres J. Cocaine abuse in older adults: an underscreened cohort. J Am Geriatr Soc 2010; 58(2): 391-2. [http://dx.doi.org/10.1111/j.1532-5415.2009.02697.x] [PMID: 20370870]

[5] Diagnostic and Statistical Manual of Mental Disorders. 5th ed., Arlington, VA: American Psychiatric Association 2013.

[6] Maxwell JC. Emerging research on methamphetamine. Curr Opin Psychiatry 2005; 18(3): 235-42. [http://dx.doi.org/10.1097/01.yco.0000165592.52811.84] [PMID: 16639146]

[7] Summary of Findings From the 2007 National Household Survey on Drug Abuse. Rockville, MD: Substance Abuse & Mental Health Services Administration, US Dept of Health & Human Services 2008.

[8] Treatment episode data set (TEDS): 1994-2004. National Admissions to Substance Abuse Treatment Services 2006.

[9] Findings from the 2004 national survey on drug use and health. Available from: http://www.drugabusestatistics.samhsa.gov/nsduh/2k4nsduh/2k4Results/2k4Results.htm#toc. 2005.

[10] National estimates of drug-related emergency department visits. Available from: http:// dawninfo.samhsa.gov. 2005.

[11] Mittleman MA, Mintzer D, Maclure M, Tofler GH, Sherwood JB, Muller JE. Triggering of myocardial infarction by cocaine. Circulation 1999; 99(21): 2737-41. [http://dx.doi.org/10.1161/01.CIR.99.21.2737] [PMID: 10351966]

[12] Wadland WC, Ferenchick GS. Medical comorbidity in addictive disorders. Psychiatr Clin North Am 2004; 27(4): 675-87. [http://dx.doi.org/10.1016/j.psc.2004.06.006] [PMID: 15550287]

[13] Castells X, Casas M, Pérez-Mañá C, Roncero C, Vidal X, Capellà D. Efficacy of psychostimulant drugs for cocaine dependence. Cochrane Database Syst Rev 2010; 2(2): CD007380. [PMID: 20166094]

[14] Mariani JJ, Levin FR. Psychostimulant treatment of cocaine dependence. Psychiatr Clin North Am 2012; 35(2): 425-39. [http://dx.doi.org/10.1016/j.psc.2012.03.012] [PMID: 22640764]

[15] Grabowski J, Rhoades H, Stotts A, *et al.* Agonist-like or antagonist-like treatment for cocaine dependence with methadone for heroin dependence: two double-blind randomized clinical trials.

Neuropsychopharmacology 2004; 29(5): 969-81.
[http://dx.doi.org/10.1038/sj.npp.1300392] [PMID: 15039761]

[16] Dackis CA, Kampman KM, Lynch KG, Pettinati HM, O'Brien CP. A double-blind, placebo-controlled trial of modafinil for cocaine dependence. Neuropsychopharmacology 2005; 30(1): 205-11.
[http://dx.doi.org/10.1038/sj.npp.1300600] [PMID: 15525998]

[17] Anderson AL, Reid MS, Li SH, *et al.* Modafinil for the treatment of cocaine dependence. Drug Alcohol Depend 2009; 104(1-2): 133-9.
[http://dx.doi.org/10.1016/j.drugalcdep.2009.04.015] [PMID: 19560290]

[18] Morgan PT, Pace-Schott E, Pittman B, Stickgold R, Malison RT. Normalizing effects of modafinil on sleep in chronic cocaine users. Am J Psychiatry 2010; 167(3): 331-40.
[http://dx.doi.org/10.1176/appi.ajp.2009.09050613] [PMID: 20080983]

[19] Shoptaw S, Heinzerling KG, Rotheram-Fuller E, *et al.* Bupropion hydrochloride *versus* placebo, in combination with cognitive behavioral therapy, for the treatment of cocaine abuse/dependence. J Addict Dis 2008; 27(1): 13-23.
[http://dx.doi.org/10.1300/J069v27n01_02] [PMID: 18551884]

[20] Shoptaw S, Heinzerling KG, Rotheram-Fuller E, *et al.* Randomized, placebo-controlled trial of bupropion for the treatment of methamphetamine dependence. Drug Alcohol Depend 2008; 96(3): 222-32.
[http://dx.doi.org/10.1016/j.drugalcdep.2008.03.010] [PMID: 18468815]

[21] Poling J, Oliveto A, Petry N, *et al.* Six-month trial of bupropion with contingency management for cocaine dependence in a methadone-maintained population. Arch Gen Psychiatry 2006; 63(2): 219-28.
[http://dx.doi.org/10.1001/archpsyc.63.2.219] [PMID: 16461866]

[22] Schmitz JM, Mooney ME, Moeller FG, Stotts AL, Green C, Grabowski J. Levodopa pharmacotherapy for cocaine dependence: choosing the optimal behavioral therapy platform. Drug Alcohol Depend 2008; 94(1-3): 142-50.
[http://dx.doi.org/10.1016/j.drugalcdep.2007.11.004] [PMID: 18164144]

[23] Brodie JD, Figueroa E, Laska EM, Dewey SL. Safety and efficacy of gamma-vinyl GABA (GVG) for the treatment of methamphetamine and/or cocaine addiction. Synapse 2005; 55(2): 122-5.
[http://dx.doi.org/10.1002/syn.20097] [PMID: 15543630]

[24] Brodie JD, Figueroa E, Dewey SL. Treating cocaine addiction: from preclinical to clinical trial experience with gamma-vinyl GABA. Synapse 2003; 50(3): 261-5.
[http://dx.doi.org/10.1002/syn.10278] [PMID: 14515344]

[25] Brodie JD, Case BG, Figueroa E, *et al.* Randomized, double-blind, placebo-controlled trial of vigabatrin for the treatment of cocaine dependence in Mexican parolees. Am J Psychiatry 2009; 166(11): 1269-77.
[http://dx.doi.org/10.1176/appi.ajp.2009.08121811] [PMID: 19651710]

[26] Reis AD, Castro LA, Faria R, Laranjeira R. Craving decrease with topiramate in outpatient treatment for cocaine dependence: an open label trial. Rev Bras Psiquiatr 2008; 30(2): 132-5.
[http://dx.doi.org/10.1590/S1516-44462008005000012] [PMID: 18470406]

[27] Kampman KM, Pettinati H, Lynch KG, *et al.* A pilot trial of topiramate for the treatment of cocaine

dependence. Drug Alcohol Depend 2004; 75(3): 233-40.
[http://dx.doi.org/10.1016/j.drugalcdep.2004.03.008] [PMID: 15283944]

[28] Mariani JJ, Pavlicova M, Bisaga A, Nunes EV, Brooks DJ, Levin FR. Extended-release mixed amphetamine salts and topiramate for cocaine dependence: a randomized controlled trial. Biol Psychiatry 2012; 72(11): 950-6.
[http://dx.doi.org/10.1016/j.biopsych.2012.05.032] [PMID: 22795453]

[29] Elkashef A, Kahn R, Yu E, *et al.* Topiramate for the treatment of methamphetamine addiction: a multi-center placebo-controlled trial. Addiction 2012; 107(7): 1297-306.
[http://dx.doi.org/10.1111/j.1360-0443.2011.03771.x] [PMID: 22221594]

[30] Pani PP, Trogu E, Vacca R, Amato L, Vecchi S, Davoli M. Disulfiram for the treatment of cocaine dependence. Cochrane Database Syst Rev 2010; (1): CD007024.
[PMID: 20091613]

[31] Haney M, Gunderson EW, Jiang H, Collins ED, Foltin RW. Cocaine-specific antibodies blunt the subjective effects of smoked cocaine in humans. Biol Psychiatry 2010; 67(1): 59-65.
[http://dx.doi.org/10.1016/j.biopsych.2009.08.031] [PMID: 19846066]

[32] Martell BA, Orson FM, Poling J, *et al.* Cocaine vaccine for the treatment of cocaine dependence in methadone-maintained patients: a randomized, double-blind, placebo-controlled efficacy trial. Arch Gen Psychiatry 2009; 66(10): 1116-23.
[http://dx.doi.org/10.1001/archgenpsychiatry.2009.128] [PMID: 19805702]

[33] Kampman KM, Dackis C, Lynch KG, *et al.* A double-blind, placebo-controlled trial of amantadine, propranolol, and their combination for the treatment of cocaine dependence in patients with severe cocaine withdrawal symptoms. Drug Alcohol Depend 2006; 85(2): 129-37.
[http://dx.doi.org/10.1016/j.drugalcdep.2006.04.002] [PMID: 16697124]

[34] Xu J, DeVito EE, Worhunsky PD, Carroll KM, Rounsaville BJ, Potenza MN. White matter integrity is associated with treatment outcome measures in cocaine dependence. Neuropsychopharmacology 2010; 35(7): 1541-9.
[http://dx.doi.org/10.1038/npp.2010.25] [PMID: 20393459]

CHAPTER 18

Tobacco Use Disorders

Frederick Petty[1,*], **James Meyer**[2] and **Vidhyalakshmi Selvaraj**[3]

[1] *Orlando VA Medical Center, Orlando, Florida, Orange City Community Based Outpatient Clinic, 2583 South Volusia Ave #300, Orange City, Florida 32763, USA*

[2] *Inroads to Recovery, 2808 N 75th ST, Omaha NE, 68134, USA*

[3] *Department of Psychiatry, Creighton University, 3528 Dodge, Omaha, NE 68131, USA*

Abstract: Tobacco is one of the most widely used drugs of abuse, and represents the single most preventable cause of death. Physicians should take every opportunity to encourage their patients who smoke to quit. Most smokers are aware of the health hazards of smoking and want to quit. Smokers also need to be made aware of the health and economic benefits of a tobacco free life. Several pharmacological agents are available to help the patient who is committed to quitting. Nicotine replacement (patch, gum, lozenge, inhaler) is the most widely used, is available over the counter, and has a success rate about twice that of placebo. Bupropion (Zyban, Wellbutrin) has a slightly higher success rate, and can be used in conjunction with nicotine replacement. Varenicline (Chantix) probably provides the best success rates. Support and self-help groups are also a very useful resource for many patients.

Keywords: Bupropion, Nicotine, Nicotine replacement, Smoking, Tobacco, Varenicline.

KEY LEARNING POINTS

1. Quitting smoking is the single most positive action that your patients can take to improve their health.
2. Smokers lose 13-14 years of life expectancy.

* **Corresponding author Frederick Petty:** Orlando VA Medical Center, Orlando, Florida Orange City Community Based Outpatient Clinic 2583 South Volusia Ave #300 Orange City, Florida 32763 USA; Tel: 386-456-2080, Fax: 407-513-9824; Email: frederick.petty2@va.gov

Subhash C. Bhatia (Ed.)

3. Medication for smoking cessation can result in over 1/3 of smokers quitting.

CLINICAL VIGNETTE

Mr. R was a 56 year old elementary school teacher, who was visiting his family physician for a routine health maintenance check up. He had a history of hypertension and dyslipidemia, both well controlled with medication. He was also about 20 pounds over his ideal body weight, but was otherwise in good health. During the clinic visit, his physician asked him if he was ready to stop smoking cigarettes. The patient was smoking about a pack of cigarettes per day, and has expressed some interest in quitting. He had stopped "cold turkey" for about a month fifteen years ago, after the birth of a child. He had also quit about ten years ago using bupropion (Wellbutrin, Zyban) plus nicotine replacement gum for several months, but returned to smoking after getting a new job and feeling under "stress." The patient had no significant other history of substance use disorder. He drank socially, never more than 6 drinks per week. He had never used marihuana, cocaine, amphetamine, or other drugs of abuse. The family physician provided brief behavioral counseling, and prescribed varenicline (Chantix), 2 mg twice a day. The patient quit successfully, and was still totally abstinent from cigarettes at a follow-up visit two months later.

RECOGNITION

Recognition of tobacco use disorder generally depends on self report. Since use of tobacco is legal, patients are less likely to give erroneous information than for illegal drugs of abuse. Also, use of tobacco does not generally have the social stigma associated with excessive alcohol use. Thus, the clinician can generally assume that a patient will be truthful about tobacco use. Excessive long term tobacco abuse can be associated with pulmonary and cardiovascular findings on the physical examination. There is a blood test which can be used to verify nicotine, serum cotinine, which is a metabolite of nicotine. However, it remains primarily a specialized or research test, and is not practical for everyday clinical use.

Tobacco used disorder is a chronic disease, and clinicians should offer every patient who smokes brief behavioral counseling. Further discussion of psychological and behavioral interventions for tobacco addiction is presented below. It should be emphasized that most (70%) smokers would like to quit.

DIAGNOSTIC ELEMENTS PRESENTED

Tobacco use disorder is usually diagnosed by self report. In cases where smokers minimize their habit, or deny it altogether, it may be helpful to have a family conference. In addition to smoking, tobacco may be used orally, as chewing tobacco or snuff.

EPIDEMIOLOGY

Tobacco is a universally available drug of abuse. The percent of Americans who smoke is now about 21%. This represents a dramatic decrease since the 1950's, when almost 50% of Americans smoked. This decrease is probably due to a number of factors, not the least of which was the Surgeon General's report on smoking and health issued in 1964. Rates of smoking are higher in developing countries, and in lower socio-economic classes. In the USA, smoking rates are the highest among Native Americans (43%); intermediate in African-Americans (23%) and Caucasians (22%); and lowest in Hispanics (15%) and Asians (10%). Marketing to women has been successful, and rates of smoking, though still lower than men, have increased over the years. Rates of smoking also vary by state, with the highest rates in Kentucky (28%) and the lowest in Utah (12%). Most (90%) smokers begin by age 21 [1].

BACKGROUND

Smoking is the most preventable cause of death and disability, and the greatest cause of excess health care costs. In the USA, 1 in 5 deaths (440,000 deaths per year) are smoking related. The largest number of these are due to lung cancer (125,000), with heart disease (82,000), and COPD (65,000) also major sources of mortality. Cigarette smoking accounts for 30% of all deaths from cancer, and 50% of long term smokers die prematurely of smoking consequences. Smokers have a 3 times greater risk of MI, a 2 times greater risk of stroke, and a 10 times greater risk of peripheral vascular disease.

Rates of smoking are higher in all mental illnesses and psychiatric disorders.

Persons with mental illness and substance use disorders are about 22% of the population, but consume 44% of the cigarettes. As relates to primary care settings, smoking in depressive disorders is about twice as high as the general population, and these patients have a greater risk of depression when quitting smoking. Rates of smoking are also 2-3 times higher in persons with substance use disorders. In fact, the greatest cause of death in persons with alcohol use disorder is smoking related illness [2].

Thus, the primary care physician should incorporate smoking cessation into her encounter with every smoking patient.

PHARMACOLOGICAL TREATMENT

Nicotine is rapidly absorbed into brain after smoking a cigarette, with peak brain levels in 10 seconds. Nicotine releases neurotransmitters (dopamine and norepinephrine) associated with its desirable effects, but tolerance rapidly develops with continuing use. When quitting, smokers must overcome psychological, behavioral, and socio-cultural associations, as well as pharmacological withdrawal. Withdrawal peaks in 7 days, and, not surprisingly, most relapsing smokers do so within the first week of quitting. Symptoms of withdrawal from nicotine can include irritability, agitation, depression, anxiety, restlessness, difficulty concentrating, insomnia, hunger, weight gain, and labile mood [3]. The clinician should have as a goal minimizing these symptoms, and reassuring the patient that they are time limited. In helping patients who smoke to quit, the clinician may consider the "5 A's".

Ask about smoking at every opportunity
Advise all smokers to quit, in a clear, strong, personalized manner
Assess patient's willingness to stop
Assist the smoker to stop
Arrange follow-up

Pharmacological treatment for smoking cessation include nicotine replacement (NRT), bupropion (Wellbutrin, Zyban), nortriptyline (Pamelor), and varenicline (Chantix). The following table lists these, along with the abstinence % at 1 year, and the odds ratio (OR) of quitting compared to placebo [4, 5].

Medication	Abstinence (%)	OR
Placebo	14	1
Bupropion SR	24	2
Nicotine Gum (6-14 weeks)	19	1.5
Nicotine Gum (>14 weeks)	26	2.2
Nicotine Lozenge	24	2.0
Nicotine Patch (6-14 weeks)	23	1.9
Varencline (1mg)	25	2.1
Varencline (2mg)	33	3.1
Nic Patch + PRN NRT (26-52 weeks)	37	3.6
Nic Patch + Bupropion	29	2.5
Nic Patch + Nortriptyline	27	2.3
Nic Patch + Nic inhaler	26	2.2

As one can see, most of these treatments have comparable results, with abstinence rates in the 20's%. Often, a patient will say that a particular treatment in the past was not successful. In cases like this, the patient should be encouraged to either try this treatment again, or be provided with another option for treatment. Following is more detailed discussion regarding the specific treatments.

Nicotine Replacement Therapy

Nicotine replacement therapy (NRT) is available as a transdermal patch, gum, lozenge, and inhaler. Except for the inhaler, these products are available without prescription, "over the counter". NRT provides the best relief of withdrawal symptoms, and provide positive reinforcement as well as relief of arousal and stress. NRT may be used in combination with other agents, and two NRT can be combined, as in patch plus gum. NRT has a very favorable side effect profile, with gastrointestinal distress occasionally seen [6].

"E-cigarettes" have recently become available, and may theoretically be useful for smoking cessation. These are stated to have only water vapor and nicotine in the inhalant. However, they may have health risks.

Whether nicotine replacement agents can themselves become dependency promoting is possible, but not researched. The long term effects of these agents is not well known, but they certainly do not have the health risk of tobacco products.

Bupropion (Zyban, Wellbutrin)

The effects of bupropion on smoking were discovered serendipitously. Bupropion is an antidepressant, with a primary mechanism of action involving the reuptake of the neurotransmitters dopamine and norepinephrine. Bupropion blocks the negative consequences of withdrawal, and attenuates the reinforcing properties of nicotine. Bupropion has a favorable side effect profile, with some patients reporting insomnia or anxiety [7].

Varenicline (Chantix)

Varenicline is a partial agonist at the nicotinic acetycholinergic receptor. Thus, varenicline releases dopamine less than nicotine, but also blocks the effects of nicotine. There has been a concern regarding neuropsychiatric symptoms as side effects of varencline, including psychosis, depression, and suicidality. Varencline may impair driving and flying. Nevertheless, these side effects have been rare in clinical use, and have not prevented wide spread use of varenicline for smoking cessation [8 - 10].

Other Agents

Nortriptyline is an antidepressant with primarily norepinephrine reuptake properties. It is an effective agent for smoking cessation, but has a worse side effect profile than bupropion, and may be considered a second line agent. Clonidine is an alpha-2 agonist, which decreases norepinephrine activity. It is not very effective for smoking cessation, but may be useful for very heavy smokers [11].

Thus, in treating smokers who wish to quit, the primary care clinician should select an agent appropriate for the patient, should encourage the patient to take the medication for an appropriate time, and provide follow-up.

Bio-psycho-social Treatment

Brief behavioral counseling is essential in helping patients quit smoking. Several points may be emphasized: "this is the single most important thing you can do to improve your health". "It's never too late to gain benefit from quitting". In this context, the "5 R's" to enhance motivation to quit smoking can be helpful:

> Relevance: why quitting is personally relevant to this patient
> Risks: what are the negative consequences of smoking
> Rewards: what are the potential benefits of stopping tobacco use (financial, health, esthetics)
> Roadblocks: what are the barriers or impediments to quitting
> Repetition: with unmotivated or relapsing patients

Sometimes it is helpful to show the patient how much they spend on cigarettes, which can easily be more than $2,000 per year, and to remind them that for this amount of money, they could afford a rather nice vacation, buy a new wardrobe, *etc*.

Nevertheless, physician advice is consistently shown to be one of the most important factors in successful smoking cessation. Starting an exercise program can help a quitting smoker's well being, and help avoid weight gain.

Common elements of practical counseling, which can be done by the primary care physician or her nursing staff during a brief office visit, include problem solving and skills training. This includes helping the patient to recognize potentially dangerous situations for smoking relapse, and developing coping skills for dealing with these. Supportive treatment involves encouraging the patient in the quit attempt, communicating caring and concern, and encouraging the patient to talk about the quitting process.

Problems often encountered by former smokers, which may be addressed in advance, include lack of support for cessation, spending time at home or at work with smokers, negative mood or depression, strong or prolonged withdrawal symptoms, weight gain, and smoking lapses.

Psychosocial Aspects of Nicotine Cessation

Regardless of how an individual chooses to quit smoking, many will relapse within the first few weeks to months after quitting. Different programs have been developed to provide education, support, and require individual accountability in assisting an individual's attempt at quitting. Availability of these programs vary considerably. In many communities, hospitals and health-oriented nonprofit organizations provide these to the public. Other sources may be employers or insurance companies providing these services to their employees or clients. Depending on the source, some of these programs are available for a small fee, others can be more expensive. Generally, most insurance plans will not reimburse the costs.

Support Groups

Support groups have been developed to assist patients by providing a support network, rather than having the patient make only an individual effort at quitting. These are generally facilitated groups following a formatted program. One of the most common is "Freedom from Smoking", a registered trademark program from the American Lung Association. Their materials are readily available for group or individual use. Groups generally begin with education and preparation for everyone in the group to make their quit attempt, with ongoing support as group members make their attempts. As group members share their successes and failures, it provides a supportive environment with members feeling more accountable for their attempts. For many participants, this provides an added incentive to help them through those first few difficult days and weeks of abstinence.

Self Help Groups

Nicotine Anonymous is an established twelve-step support group utilizing the same twelve steps as the original twelve step group, Alcoholics Anonymous, with the twelve steps adapted slightly to emphasize the control that nicotine has over the lives of the smoker. In most areas, local meetings are not common, with larger metropolitan areas having occasional meetings scheduled. The national organization advertises they are quite eager to help interested individuals in establishing local meetings in any area. For patients with a history of drug or alcohol recovery, most find applying their twelve step program to tobacco cessation a very natural step and this should be encouraged. Using online access to attend Nicotine Anonymous meetings is likely the easiest way to find support from this organization as there are several online meetings in various chatrooms available daily.

Telephone Quitlines

As pressure has mounted on individual states to provide more services to help smokers quit smoking, telephone quitlines have become popular as an effective, economical, way of reaching the greatest number of smokers and providing a service that is meaningful. This pressure has come as most of the individual states have received a considerable amount of money from the major tobacco companies since 1998, when the Tobacco Master Settlement Agreement was implemented. Little of this funding has been spent to actually curb tobacco use, and most state Medicaid plans will not even reimburse treatment for smoking cessation. At the present time, expert counseling is available to the patient by calling a toll-free number. Bilingual services are available sixteen hours a day with an unlimited number of sessions available with a trained counselor. A personal quit plan will be established. Some states will provide free nicotine replacement in the form of nicotine patches or gum. Referral can be made to other local programs in the caller's area. At the present time, this service is available nationwide at 1-80--QUIT NOW. Numerous studies show that the more support a smoker has available in their attempt at quitting, the more likely they are to succeed. As this service is either funded by the major tobacco companies through the Tobacco Master Settlement Agreement or the individual states with tobacco excise taxes, smokers can be encouraged to take advantage of this very helpful means of support as a service they have already paid for.

Many smokers when faced with either wanting to quit, or needing to quit, will feel quite overwhelmed. Many will truly need a referral to some form of psychosocial support to have any chance at succeeding and all will improve their chances of success with such a referral.

Treatment Outcome as it Relates to the Vignette

Mr. R. was able to quit smoking successfully, but should be provided additional follow-up and counseling, as well as encouragement.

SUMMARY

- Tobacco smoking is harmful and addictive.
- All smokers should be counseled to quit, and offered help with quitting.
- Benefits (financial, health, physical, psychological) of smoking cessation should be emphasized.
- Medications can help with smoking cessation.

TOBACCO USE DISORDER: PATIENT EDUCATION SHEET

What is it?

Tobacco is a leaf which is usually used by smoking, generally in cigarettes. The active ingredient in tobacco is nicotine.

Common Symptoms of Intoxication, Withdrawal, and Dependence

Smoking usually causes a sensation of mental alertness. Persons who are dependent on tobacco can experience symptoms of withdrawal if they do not smoke frequently, including nervousness, anxiety, irritability, trouble concentrating, depression, anger, hunger, and agitation. Smoking relieves these symptoms.

Medical Complications

Smoking is the most preventable cause of death and disability. 50% of long term smokers die prematurely of smoking causes. Smokers lose 13-14 years of life expectancy. Common medical consequences of smoking include lung cancer, chronic obstructive pulmonary disease, heart disease, stroke, and other cancers.

Psychiatric Complications

Nicotine withdrawal can be associated with anxiety and depression. In some cases, these conditions may need treatment.

How is it Treated?

Medications

Three medications are approved for smoking cessation: nicotine replacement (Nicorette, Habitrol, gum, patch, lozenge); bupropion (Wellbutrin, Zyban); varenicline (Chantix). Abstinence rates vary with medication treatment, with most in the 20% range. These medications have minimal side effects. Nicotine may cause nausea and gastric upset. Bupropion can cause restlessness and insomnia. Varenicline, in rare cases, may cause depression, psychosis, and suicidal thoughts. Failure to quit on one medication does not mean that the smoker cannot quit successfully with another. Talk to your doctor about a quit plan and about which medication is best for you.

Non-pharmacological

Support groups and self help are available in most cities.

Do's and Don'ts

When you make the decision to quit, commit yourself to total freedom from tobacco. Most relapses in persons who quit smoking are due to thinking they can smoke "just one", only to rapidly returning to previous smoking patterns. Smokers who are trying to quit have may have problems with lack of support, mild depression, withdrawal symptoms, weight gain, or smoking lapses. Often several attempts at quitting are needed before success is achieved. Stopping smoking is the single most important thing smokers can do for their health. It is never too late to quit. Most smokers would like to quit. Almost all former smokers feel physically and psychologically better, and are glad they quit.

Long-term Outcomes

The long term consequences of smoking are never positive. Even persons who do not develop cancer inevitably have problems with chronic bronchitis and emphysema.

Resources

www.smokefree.gov/

www.nlm.nih.gov/medlineplus/quittingsmoking.html

www.cancer.org/Healthy/.../GuidetoQuittingSmoking/index

CONFLICT OF INTEREST

The authors confirm that they have no conflict of interest to declare for this publication.

ACKNOWLEDGEMENTS

Declared none.

REFERENCES

[1] U. S. Public Health Service Report. A clinical practice guideline for treating tobacco use and dependence: 2008 update. Am J Prev Med 2008; 35(2): 158-76. [http://dx.doi.org/10.1016/j.amepre.2008.04.009] [PMID: 18617085]

[2] Mundey K. An appraisal of smoking cessation aids. Curr Opin Pulm Med 2009; 15(2): 105-12. [http://dx.doi.org/10.1097/MCP.0b013e328321862e] [PMID: 19532024]

[3] Benowitz NL. Pharmacology of nicotine: addiction, smoking-induced disease, and therapeutics. Annu Rev Pharmacol Toxicol 2009; 49: 57-71. [http://dx.doi.org/10.1146/annurev.pharmtox.48.113006.094742] [PMID: 18834313]

[4] Eisenberg MJ, Filion KB, Yavin D, *et al.* Pharmacotherapies for smoking cessation: a meta-analysis of randomized controlled trials. CMAJ 2008; 179(2): 135-44. [http://dx.doi.org/10.1503/cmaj.070256] [PMID: 18625984]

[5] VHA Pharmacy Benefits Management Services. Recommendations for use of combination therapy in tobacco use cessation. Available from: http://www.pbm.va.gov 2009.

[6] Frishman WH. Smoking cessation pharmacotherapy. Ther Adv Cardiovasc Dis 2009; 3(4): 287-308. [http://dx.doi.org/10.1177/1753944709335754] [PMID: 19491139]

[7] Carrozzi L, Pistelli F, Viegi G. Pharmacotherapy for smoking cessation. Ther Adv Respir Dis 2008; 2(5): 301-17. [http://dx.doi.org/10.1177/1753465808096136] [PMID: 19124379]

[8] Galanti LM. Tobacco smoking cessation management: integrating varenicline in current practice. Vasc Health Risk Manag 2008; 4(4): 837-45. [PMID: 19066000]

[9] Garrison GD, Dugan SE. Varenicline: a first-line treatment option for smoking cessation. Clin Ther 2009; 31(3): 463-91.
[http://dx.doi.org/10.1016/j.clinthera.2009.03.021] [PMID: 19393839]

[10] Hays JT, Ebbert JO. Varenicline for tobacco dependence. N Engl J Med 2008; 359(19): 2018-24.
[http://dx.doi.org/10.1056/NEJMct0800146] [PMID: 18987369]

[11] Ebbert JO. Emerging drugs for the treatment of tobacco dependence. Expert Opin Emerg Drugs 2009; 14(1): 23-32.
[http://dx.doi.org/10.1517/14728210802623874] [PMID: 19278367]

CHAPTER 19

Non-Substance-Related Addictive Disorders

Subhash C. Bhatia[1,*] and **Shashi K. Bhatia**[2]

[1] *Department of Psychiatry, Mental Health and Behavioral Sciences, Creighton University; Department VA Nebraska- Western Iowa Health Care System 4101 Woolworth Ave Omaha, NE 68105, USA*

[2] *Departments of Psychiatry and Pediatrics, Division of Child and Adolescent Psychiatry, Creighton University, 3528 Dodge Omaha, NE 68131, USA*

Abstract: Historically, since ancient times mankind around the globe has resorted to gambling behavior in one or other form, there is no specific cause for gambling addiction. Like other addictions genetic, biological, psychological and environmental causes play a part. Often competitive workaholics are drawn to gambling. Drugs like levodopa for parkinsonism may increase gambling behavior. Gambling is more common in younger individuals with no difference between sexes. Gambling has similar reward pathways as for other addictions and has impulsive and compulsive quality. These individuals show preoccupation with gambling, seek thrill from it, hide or lie about losses and at times experience remorse or guilt and try unsuccessfully to cut down and often chase their losses with a hope to "hit a big jackpot". Diagnosis is based on DSM-5 criteria. Certain scales can be used to assess its severity. There are no known proven preventive strategies for gambling. Also there are no approved pharmacological interventions, however research favors therapeutic value of SSRIs, mood stabilizers and opiate antagonists . Like for other addictions gambling and related disorders also benefit from motivational enhancement, individual, group, couple and family therapies as well as self-help groups like Gambling Anonymous (GA).

Keywords: Card game gambling, Casino gambling, Cockfight, Compulsive gambling, Dogfight betting, Horse race betting, Internet gaming and gambling, Lottery betting, Pathological gambling, Problem gambling, Slot machine gambling, Sports betting, Wagering.

[*] **Corresponding author Subhash C. Bhatia:** Department of Psychiatry, Mental Health and Behavioral Sciences, Creighton University; Department VA Nebraska- Western Iowa Health Care System 4101 Woolworth Ave Omaha, NE 68105, USA; Tel: (402) 995-4315; Fax: (402) 995-4240; Email: sub55@cox.net

KEY LEARNING POINTS

1. Non-Substance-Related Addictive Disorders in literature also described as Behavioral Addictions or "Soft Addictions". Some of the examples of such addictions are: gambling, internet, sex, food, exercise, pornography and shopping *etc*.
2. Like substances these additive behaviors are persistent, repetitive, compulsive and problematic. These continue despite negative social, legal and occupational consequences.
3. Non- substance related addictions like substance related addictions are also mediated through brain reward circuits.
4. Because of available research data about epidemiology, clinical course and biological factors Gambling Disorder is included in DSM-5 chapter on addictive disorder. However Internet Gaming Disorder lacks such a data and therefore in DSM-5 it is part of the section on Conditions for Further Study.
5. For gambling disorder pharmacological interventions with SSRIs and opioid antagonists and psychological interventions with behavioral and cognitive behavioral therapy have data for efficacy.

CLINICAL VIGNETTE

Mr. A is a 36 year old Caucasian male a 7th grade mathematics teacher came with his wife, a registered nurse with symptoms of depression with suicidal intent and plan. He was also not able to function well at work. He admitted to craving about going to casino with a confidence that he will figure out a way to recuperate his losses. He stated that he wanted to die through a planned motor vehicle accident to mimic an accidental death in order for his family receiving life insurance benefits to cover his gambling debts as well as other financial obligations.

History revealed that for the last 10 years patient has been gambling excessively. He stated that at least 2 to 3 times a week he was either at casinos or horse race track. During this period, the patient has gambled away most of his savings including funds set aside for education of his 7 year old son. He recently has a warrant against him for arrest for forging checks. His wife discovered notices from the bank for insufficient funds and financial penalties related to that. Mrs. A confronted her husband many a times and every time he had a different excuse or different lie. Recently in response to these confrontations Mr. A displayed remorse and guilt and at times was able to cut down on his gambling for short periods. A few times he also made contact with 12-step Gamblers Anonymous (GA). His wife stated that she was "fed up" with her husband's gambling behavior and had contacted a divorce attorney to file for separation.

In addition to Gambling Disorder, Mr. A was diagnosed to have major depression of moderate severity and was admitted to residential rehabilitation gambling addiction treatment program. Initially patient was in denial and felt that he is endowed with a gift to win and "it was just a matter of time for a big win and he will be able to compensate his losses". Early on the couple therapy sessions were stormy. With non confrontational supportive and empathic approach and motivational enhancement therapy in about 3 weeks he acknowledged some need for treatment and started to invest in his own recovery. He was prescribed an antidepressant sertraline 50 mg a daily in the morning and trazodone 100 mg at bed time. He also received cognitive behavioral therapy. His wife also decided to engage in couple therapy. While in the program, his depression gradually improved but he struggled with making a change in his gambling mind set. Patient was discharged from the residential rehabilitation program after a month. Soon after that he returned to work as a teacher. Patient continued outpatient cognitive behavioral therapy and antidepressant medication as well as participated in GA meetings. He also retained a sponsor. During a 12 month follow up period, patient denied have craving to return to casinos and was getting along better with his wife and colleagues at school. He also developed a restitution plan to retire his gambling debt.

Discussion of Vignette

This patient meets the DSM-5 diagnostic criteria for both gambling and major depressive disorder. This better outcome is possible because of better understanding of psychopathology and neurobiology of gambling and related disorders. The success of treatment in this patient was due to multimodal intervention; like motivation enhancement, individual, couple, pharmacotherapy and participation in self-help group. These interventions are similar to those used for other addictive disorders. Selective serotonin reuptake inhibitor (SSRI) like sertraline may have a dual therapeutic role both for the treatment of depression as well as gambling behavior since increase serotonergic activity in the brain also promotes anti impulsive behavior.

BACKGROUND

Non-substance-related addictions or behavioral addictions are similar to chemical addictions. In both, patients engage in compulsive, repetitive out of control behaviors to seek excitement. In DSM IV –TR the pathological gambling was classified under Impulse Control Disorders Not Elsewhere Classified [1]. In International Statistical Classification of Diseases and Related Health Problems (ICD- 10) pathological gambling, pathological fire setting, pathological stealing and trichotillomania are classified under "Habit and Impulse Disorders" "characterized by repeated acts that have no clear rational motivation, cannot be controlled by the patient and usually harmful interests of self and others". Patient reports that the behavior is associated with "impulses to action" [2]. In DSM -5 because of research evidence Gambling Disorder is included in chapter on addictive disorder. However other non-substance related addictions due to lack of strong research evidence like Internet Gaming Disorder is included in Conditions for Further Study [3].

Historically since ancient times mankind has resorted to gambling behavior in one or other form. Around the world the gambling and opportunities like online casinos, lotteries, sports, horse tracks, card games and slot machine gambling are in abundance. In US about 3 to 5 percent of population has problem gambling and about 1 percent population meet the criteria for pathological gambling. It is more common in males than females also in females' onset is later. A modal patient for this disorder is a Caucasian male in his 30s from middle to upper socioeconomic class with materialistic orientation.

Currently gambling poses a significant public health problem in US and around the globe.

NEUROBIOLOGY

There are similarities between neurobiology and genetics of drug and nondrug related addictions. In healthy brain there is a satiety related feedback to the regions of brain responsible for limiting specific behaviors. American Society of Addiction Medicine in 2011 described "addiction as a primary chronic disease of brain reward, motivation, memory and related circuits" and further stated that addiction is not solely substance dependence. As a result behavioral addictions are included in section on addictive disorders [4, 5]. Like cravings in alcoholics allele of dopamine-2 receptor gene plays a part in addictive disorder [6]. Family history of pathological gamblers show higher rate of substance use disorder specially alcoholism and depressive disorders. Amygdala is associated with emotional memory and cue driven behaviors [7 - 9]. Dysfunction of ventro-medial prefrontal cortex circuitry is the cause for impulsivity expressed as sense of urgency, lack of evaluative and rational decision making processes. Such dysfunction impairs prefrontal "brake system" resulting in repetitive impulsive maladaptive behaviors. Prefrontal cortex, amygdala, mesocorticolimbic system associated with reward, dysfunctional feedback and neuroplasticity play a part in addictive processes [10 - 12]. Functional neuroimaging studies in drug and nondrug related addictions for instance, in gambling shows similarity in activation in certain brain regions [13]. Moreover therapeutic interventions both for drug and nondrug addictive behavior are similar. Studies show that addictive behaviors and some psychiatric disorders like mood, personality, impulse control and attention deficit are often comorbid [14] like was the case in our patient for major depression.

ASSESSMENT

This requires assessment of readiness for change, co-occurring mental or substance use disorder, severity of gambling problem and risk of self-harm. There are screening instruments like South Oaks Gambling Screen (SOGS) [15], Massachusetts Gambling Screen (MAGS) [16]; World Health Organization: Composite International Diagnostic Interview [17]. DSM-5 diagnostic criteria (3) are available for diagnosis of gambling disorder. This includes 9 diagnostic criteria for gambling disorder. The severity of this disorder is determined by the number of symptoms present *i.e.* 4-5 symptoms for mild, 6-7 for moderate and 8-9 for severe.

INTERNET GAMING DISORDER

This is another non-substance-related and addictive disorder. Due to inadequate research data, in DSM-5 this disorder is included in section on Conditions for Further Study [3] on pages 795-798. In literature this is also referred to as Internet use disorder, internet addiction, internet addiction disorder, gaming addiction *etc.* This disorder has higher prevalence among Asian population [3].

TREATMENT CONSIDERATIONS

Because of ubiquity of gambling behavior a public policy consideration is important. In this section treatment of only gambling disorders will be discussed. Patients with this disorder, unless associated with imminent danger to self or others, can be safely treated in residential treatment settings, in partial hospital or as outpatients. Repeated failure of lesser restrictive treatment environment of care may require more intense level of care. The co-occurring psychiatric disorders require appropriate treatment [18] based on their severity with or without danger to self or others.

PHARMACOLOGICAL INTERVENTIONS

There are no FDA-approved medications for the treatment of gambling disorders. Psychopharmacological research in management of this disorder show that antidepressants, mood stabilizers, opioid antagonists may be of value in treatment of gambling disorder.

SSRIs play a role in the management of anxiety, depression, obsessive compulsive, and impulsive pattern of addictive behavior.

Double-blind placebo controlled studies with opioid antagonist nalmefene showed that these reduce intense urge or carving to gamble in a fashion similar to alcoholics [19]. The use of naltrexone is approved for alcohol use disorder. Like in alcoholics opiate antagonists may also reduce pleasurable effects and craving to gamble. With normal liver functions start with a dose of 25 mg a day for two days followed by 50 mg a day there after.

Mood stabilizers like lithium and valproic acid are of value if gambling is associated with bipolar disorder.

Recently a glutamate-modulator N-acetyl cysteine has been noted to reduce urges to gamble [19].

Psychological Interventions

Strength of evidence for various psychosocial interventions for gambling disorder is strong for Cognitive Behavior Therapy (CBT) and Behavioral Therapy; moderate for Relapse Prevention and weak for psychodynamic psychotherapy, aversion therapy, 12-step GA and self-exclusion from casinos or gambling places [20].

1. Behavioral therapy: Aversion is rarely used. However individual stimulus control and cue exposure with response prevention, systematic imaginal desensitization to include imaginal relaxation and imaginal desensitization are effective therapies.
2. Self-exclusion is arranging one's own debarment from gambling facilities for specified period of time on a voluntary basis.
3. CBT has a strong strength of evidence for effectiveness. This requires identification of core cognitive distortions and errors associated with gambling *i.e.* illusion of control over gambling outcome, feeling of omnipotent skill to beat odds. These distortions need to be challenged with reality based data. Cognitive restructuring directed toward changing distorted thoughts, beliefs and attitudes related to gambling and winning as well as developing self-efficaciousness.
4. Relapse prevention requires assessment of stages of change, movement from action to maintenance phase. In addition having patent recognize high risk situations for gambling and developing prevention and coping strategies

Social Interventions

1. Social and coping skills, problem solving skills, psychoeducation, learning to manage impulse to gamble, planning to fill the time utilized by gambling with leisure and enjoyable hobbies.
2. Financial counseling is to help individuals to learn budgeting, develop payment plan. The financial counseling should be available to individuals with gambling problems as well as for those affected by gambling.
3. GA a 12-step is a spirituality-based self-help groups without professional facilitation. This is frequently a part of after care plan.

SUMMARY

Non-substance-related and addictive disorders have similar neurobiological underpinning as other addictive disorders. Except for gambling disorder the research data for other behavioral addictions is rather inadequate. That is why internet gaming disorder is included in the DSM-5 section on Conditions for Further Study. There are no approved pharmacological interventions for gambling disorder; however available research data favors therapeutic value of SSRIs, mood stabilizers and opiate antagonists. Like for other addictions in gambling disorder motivational enhancement, individual, group, couple and family therapies as well as self-help groups have proven value. Despite that small percentage of patients continue to struggle because of high relapse rate.

NON-SUBSTANCE-RELATED AND ADDICTIVE DISORDERS (NSRADS) - PATIENT EDUCATION SHEET

What are NSRADs?

These disorders are similar to other addictive disorders. These are also called behavioral addictions. Some of the example of such addictions relate to behaviors associated with gambling, sex, pornography, videogames, internet, food, work, exercise, shopping *etc.*

Why these Behaviors are Considered Disorders?

Just like with drug addictions vulnerable individuals with behavioral addictions show failure to control these behaviors, compulsively repeat these behaviors despite negative consequences related to personal, social, family, occupation and finances.

What are the Symptoms of NSRADs?

The symptoms are similar to drug related addictions like persistent and recurrent engagement of these behaviors, are source of excitement or "high", individuals are unsuccessful in controlling these behaviors despite multiple attempts to reduce or stop, crave to reengage in these behaviors, experience social, educational, occupational and financial problems and may even show tolerance and withdrawal and that these are not caused by other mental disorder like bipolar disorder or major depression.

Are there any Medications to Treat NSRADs?

There are no FDA approved medications. However drugs from Prozac family and drugs approved for use to reduce carving in alcoholics to like an opiate antagonist naltrexone are promising.

What Other Treatments are Recommended to Treat NDRADs?

Individual, family, couple or group talk therapy and spiritually-based self-help groups similar to Alcoholic Anonymous (AA) for example Gamblers Anonymous (GA)for gambling addiction, social skills training, financial counseling and voluntary self-exclusion from gambling facilities.

The link for GA is: www.gamblersanonymous.org.

CONFLICT OF INTEREST

The authors confirm that they have no conflict of interest to declare for this publication.

ACKNOWLEDGEMENTS

Declared none.

REFERENCES

[1] American Psychiatric Association. Diagnostic and Statistical Manual of Mental disorders. Fourth Edition, Text Revision., Washington, DC: American Psychiatric Association 2000.

[2] World Health Organization. International classification of diseases and related health problems, 10th revision (ICD-10).. Geneva: World Health Organization 1992.

[3] American Psychiatric Association. Diagnostic and statistical manual of mental disorders. 5th ed., Arlington, VA: American Psychiatric Association 2013.

[4] American Society of Addiction Medicine. Public Policy Statement: Definition of Addiction. 2011. Available from: http://www.asam.org/Definitionofaddiction-LongVersion.html

[5] American Society of Addiction Medicine. Public Policy Statement: Definition of Addiction: Frequently asked questions. 2011. Available from: http://www.asam.org/pdf/Advocacy/20110816_Defo-Addiction-FAQs.pdf

[6] Goodman A. Neurobiology of addiction. An integrative review. Biochem Pharmacol 2008; 75(1): 266-322.
[http://dx.doi.org/10.1016/j.bcp.2007.07.030] [PMID: 17764663]

[7] Brewer JA, Potenza MN. The neurobiology and genetics of impulse control disorders: relationships to drug addictions. Biochem Pharmacol 2008; 75(1): 63-75.
[http://dx.doi.org/10.1016/j.bcp.2007.06.043] [PMID: 17719013]

[8] Girault J-A, Greengard P. The neurobiology of dopamine signaling. Arch Neurol 2004; 61(5): 641-4.
[http://dx.doi.org/10.1001/archneur.61.5.641] [PMID: 15148138]

[9] Di Chiara G, Bassareo V. Reward system and addiction: what dopamine does and doesn't do. Curr Opin Pharmacol 2007; 7(1): 69-76.
[http://dx.doi.org/10.1016/j.coph.2006.11.003] [PMID: 17174602]

[10] Kalivas PW, O'Brien C. Drug addiction as a pathology of staged neuroplasticity. Neuropsychopharmacology 2008; 33(1): 166-80.
[http://dx.doi.org/10.1038/sj.npp.1301564] [PMID: 17805308]

[11] Koob GF, Volkow ND. Neurocircuitry of addiction. Neuropsychopharmacology 2010; 35(1): 217-38.
[http://dx.doi.org/10.1038/npp.2009.110] [PMID: 19710631]

[12] Olsen CM. Natural rewards, neuroplasticity, and non-drug addictions. Neuropharmacology 2011; 61(7): 1109-22.
[http://dx.doi.org/10.1016/j.neuropharm.2011.03.010] [PMID: 21459101]

[13] Breiter HC, Aharon I, Kahneman D, Dale A, Shizgal P. Functional imaging of neural responses to expectancy and experience of monetary gains and losses. Neuron 2001; 30(2): 619-39.
[http://dx.doi.org/10.1016/S0896-6273(01)00303-8] [PMID: 11395019]

[14] Petry NM, Stinson FS, Grant BF. Comorbidity of DSM-IV pathological gambling and other psychiatric disorders: results from the National Epidemiologic Survey on Alcohol and Related Conditions. J Clin Psychiatry 2005; 66(5): 564-74.
[http://dx.doi.org/10.4088/JCP.v66n0504] [PMID: 15889941]

[15] Lesieur HR, Blume SB. The South Oaks Gambling Screen (SOGS): a new instrument for the

identification of pathological gamblers. Am J Psychiatry 1987; 144(9): 1184-8. [http://dx.doi.org/10.1176/ajp.144.9.1184] [PMID: 3631315]

[16] Shaffer HJ, Labrie R, Scanlan KM, Cummings TN. Pathological gambling among adolescents: Massachusetts Gambling Screen (MAGS). J Gambl Stud 1994; 10(4): 339-62. [http://dx.doi.org/10.1007/BF02104901] [PMID: 24234969]

[17] Composite International Diagnostic Interview, Version 21. Geneva: World Health Organization 1993.

[18] Hodgins DC, Stea JN, Grant JE. Gambling disorders. Lancet 2011; 378(9806): 1874-84. [http://dx.doi.org/10.1016/S0140-6736(10)62185-X] [PMID: 21600645]

[19] Grant JE, Kim SW, Odlaug BL. N-acetyl cysteine, a glutamate-modulating agent, in the treatment of pathological gambling: a pilot study. Biol Psychiatry 2007; 62(6): 652-7. [http://dx.doi.org/10.1016/j.biopsych.2006.11.021] [PMID: 17445781]

[20] Korn DA, Shaffer HJ. Massachusetts Department of Public Health's Practice Guidelines for Treating Gambling-Related Problems: An Evidenced-based Guide for Clinicians. Council on Compulsive Gambling 2004. Available from: htttp://www.masscompulsivegambling.org/stuff/contentmgr/files/fc47f00-95c626d286284aeec72d85

CHAPTER 20

Cognitive-Behavioral Therapy and Other Psychosocial Interventions for Substance Use Disorders

Aly Hassan[1,*], **Shashi K. Bhatia**[2] and **Subhash C. Bhatia**[3,4]

[1] *Phoenix VA Health Care System, Department of Psychiatry, University of Arizona, Phoenix College of Medicine, Gilbert VA Clinic, 3285 S Val Vista Drive, Gilbert AZ 85925, USA*

[2] *Departments of Psychiatry and Pediatrics, Division of Child and Adolescent Psychiatry, Creighton University, 3528 Dodge Omaha, NE 68131, USA*

[3] *Department of Psychiatry, Mental Health and Behavioral Sciences, Creighton University*

[4] *Department VA Nebraska- Western Iowa Health Care System 4101 Woolworth Ave Omaha, NE 68105, USA*

Abstract: The effectiveness of psychosocial evidenced-based behavioral interventions for substance and non-substance related disorders are comparable to their effectiveness for other psychiatric disorders . Cognitive behavioral therapy addresses the negative and dysfunctional thoughts and emotions related to these disorders and their reinforcing effects. This also helps develop cognitive skills to deal with cue driven craving leading to reengagement in addictive behaviors. Contingency management uses tangible rewards to support addiction free life style evidenced by negative drug screen participation in individual and group therapy. Behavioral self-control promotes goal setting and self-monitoring for harm reduction. Self-help 12-step programs promote acceptance, surrender to a higher power and self-governance through utilization of support from AA fellowship community. Motivational enhancement therapy is to help individuals to move higher on stages of change and to promote self-efficacy. Solution-based therapy helps patients find solutions while reinforcing their successes in solving those problems. All these therapies with or without pharmacotherapy have value in achieving addiction free life style.

* **Corresponding author Aly Hassan:** Phoenix VA Health Care System, Department of Psychiatry, University of Arizona, Phoenix College of Medicine, Gilbert VA Clinic, 3285 S Val Vista Drive, Gilbert AZ 85925, USA; Tel/Fax: (480)397-2830/(480)825-7282; Email: aly.hassan@va.gov

Subhash C. Bhatia (Ed.)

Keywords: AA, Behavioral self-control training (BSCT), CA, Cognitive-Behavioral Therapy (CBT), Contingency management (CM), GA, Motivational Enhancement Therapy (MET), NA, Relapse Prevention (RP), Voucher-based reinforcement (VBR).

KEY LEARNING POINTS

1. Cognitive Behavioral Therapy (CBT) for substance use disorder is based on the theory that substance and non-substance related maladaptive behaviors and dysfunctional emotions are learned through their powerfully reinforcing effects.
2. Cognitive strategy may include appreciating consequences of continued use, confronting thoughts to reuse substances and developing skills to discontinue such a use.
3. CBT can be utilized as an individual, couple, family or group approach in a variety of treatment settings such as acute inpatient, therapeutic community, residential programs or outpatient visits.
4. CBT includes social and coping skills training to enhance the person's capacity to verbally and nonverbally communicate, develop empathy and maintain relationships, and to be assertive.
5. CBT aids in identifying triggers and cravings, creating skills to deal with such, as well as crafting relapse prevention strategies.
6. Other psychosocial interventions include Motivation Enhancement Therapy (MET), Contingency Management (CM), and Relapse Prevention (RP) which assist in training to recognize and deal with cues to reuse.
7. Twelve-Step self-help programs like Alcoholics Anonymous (AA), Narcotics Anonymous (NA), Cocaine Anonymous (CA), and programs for non-substance related disorders like Gamblers Anonymous (GA) involve acceptance, surrender to a higher power, and self-governance.

PSYCHO-SOCIAL INTERVENTIONS FOR SUBSTANCE USE DISORDERS

"I tried to quit smoking many times, It won't work as long as my wife continues to smoke"

"Doctor I am at a point in where I am not looking for highs any more, I just

don't want to go through the withdrawal"

"For years I enjoyed my rolling joints, Since I stopped I don't know what to do with my fingers. I never thought that this will be a problem"

"Since I stopped drinking I stay home, All my friends drink, I know that it is too risky to go out with them"

These are real statements from real patients describing the complex bio-psychosocial interplay in substance use disorders, classical conditioning, positive and negative reinforcement, social learning, socio-economic status, access to care and cultural values are all important variables that influence development, complications and treatment outcomes of addictions.

The first part of the chapter reviews evidence based psychosocial treatment Approaches while the second part is dedicated to the American society of Addiction medicine placement criteria, A standardized tool to assess substance use needs and the corresponding treatment level.

Screening, Brief Interventions and Referral to Treatment

A brief intervention targeting harmful and risky use, that did not reach addiction threshold, the effectiveness of the intervention and the relatively limited cost and time resources, make it an appropriate tool in Primary care and ER settings. The duration may vary from 5-30 minutes. The goal of the intervention is to assess hazardous or harmful substance use, followed by a brief discussion, education and advice . The Acronym "FRAMES" refers to the components of the intervention. FRAMES:- Feedback, Responsibility, Advice, Menu of options, Empathy and Self efficacy (confidence for change).

Feedback

After performing assessment of substance use problems . Providing Feedback about the risks associated with current use risks and harms. It is useful to provide comparisons between the patient's pattern of use *vs.* average patterns in the population and problem patterns.

Responsibility

Communicating a message that the provider acknowledges that the patient always controls his own choices regarding the use behaviors

> *"it is my responsibility to provide you with this information to ensure that you know the risks, but I recognize that your life choices are up to you and no one else's business"*

Advice

Shedding light and Increasing the patients awareness of the patterns of substance use that may lead to new health or other problems or worsen the already existing problems.

Communicating a message about the value of cutting down or stopping substance use in improving health or reduce the risk of future problems may be valuable in fostering behavioral changes.

Menu of Alternative Change Options

Provide a list of choices that may assist the patient with the goal of changing patterns of harmful use.

- Keeping a diary of substance consumption (where, when, how much, who with, why).
- Assist patients in preparing guidelines regarding their use of the substance.
- Identifying high risk triggers and determine strategies to address them.
- Identifying alternative activities that distract from substance use – (sports, hobbies, *etc.*).
- Identify persons that can provide a supportive environment in the patient's goals
- Provide information and educational materials, provide referrals to professional and specialized care and self-help resources.

Empathy

An accepting attitude, with warm reflective pattern of communication is more successful than a directive condemning style of relating. Patients presenting with hazardous substance use have reasons to maintain their current pattern of use. Understanding their reasons and circumstances (not justifying it) in a supportive environment is an essential step.

Self-efficacy (Confidence)

Failure to believe in one's capacity to change is an obstacle towards addressing hazardous use, reframing what a patient perceives as a failure into a partial success will promote confidence into a lasting change.

-"I tried to stop smoking many times, but It did not work out". This can be reframed as:
-"I see in the records that you stopped smoking several time for periods ranging from 3 months to one week in the last ten years. Quitting smoking is a challenging matter, research says that the more attempts even with brief successes will eventually lead to a lasting outcome, I see that you were able to take the decision and pursue it for a period of time"

SELF HELP

I. Alcoholic Anonymous, and other 12 Steps Self-help Groups

Alcoholic Anonymous and other 12 steps groups are fellowship program where group members share experiences and provide strength and hope to help each other reach recovery with mutual help being the main drive to achieve behavioral, spiritual and cognitive changes. They are widely distributed and easily accessible with no cost involved, making it a significant asset in addressing substance use problems not only in the US but internationally. Alcoholic anonymous approach regards addiction as a relapsing problem, The goal should be complete abstinence.

A central value in the AA philosophy is to acknowledge to themselves (and others) the harm that substance abuse caused. Another important value is to recognize that as individuals they are powerless regarding their use and surrender to a higher power to achieve their recovery, we found in our practice that for many, the AA spiritual dimension is an asset, however for a subset of patients it raises questions that prevent them from identifying with the group [1 - 3].

Members of AA sequentially go through the following 12 steps:

1. We admitted we were powerless over alcohol—that our lives had become unmanageable.
2. Came to believe that a power greater than ourselves could restore us to sanity.
3. Made a decision to turn our will and our lives over to the care of God as we understood Him.
4. Made a searching and fearless moral inventory of ourselves.
5. Admitted to God, to ourselves, and to another human being the exact nature of our wrongs.
6. Were entirely ready to have God remove all these defects of character.
7. Humbly asked Him to remove our shortcomings.
8. Made a list of all persons we had harmed, and became willing to make amends to them all.
9. Made direct amends to such people wherever possible, except when to do so would injure them or others.
10. Continued to take personal inventory, and when we were wrong, promptly admitted it.
11. Sought through prayer and meditation to improve our conscious contact with God as we understood Him, praying only for knowledge of His will for us and the power to carry that out.
12. Having had a spiritual awakening as the result of these steps, we tried to carry this message to alcoholics, and to practice these principles in all our affairs.

Similar programs for other substances and behavioral addictions include Narcotic Anonymous (NA), Cocaine Anonymous (CA), Gamblers Anonymous (GA), Crystal-Meth Anonymous (CMA), Overeaters Anonymous (OA), They are all modeled after the AA above mentioned principals.

Research Findings comparing AA to other substance abuse treatment modalities have been mixed (Project Matching Alcoholism Treatment to Client Heterogeneity (MATCH)) showed that a 12-step program for alcohol use problems is comparable to the outcomes of CBT and motivational enhancement interventions, On the other hand a Cochrane review in 2009, the review of 8 studies did not demonstrate a clear outcome in favor of the 12 steps facilitation programs in alcohol use disorders.

II. Smart Recovery (Self-Management and Recovery Training)

Offers an approach to addiction recovery that is secular with no reference to a higher power. The approach identifies four Areas: Building motivation, Coping with urges, Problem solving (Manage thoughts, feelings, and behaviors and Life style balance (finding equilibrium between) momentary and enduring satisfactions).

SMART drives its model from heavily researched psychological interventions in cognitive behavioral therapy, and motivational interviewing.

The program is based on group meetings that are free, the encounters are intended to be informational as well as supportive. They are led by volunteer facilitators with the assistance of volunteer recovery professionals called Volunteer Advisors

COGNITIVE BEHAVIORAL THERAPIES

Cognitive Behavioral Therapies for substance use disorders include interventions based on classical learning theories (Classical, operant conditioning and social learning) and cognitive restructuring.

Cognitive strategies identify and correct (restructure) automatic dysfunctional patterns of thinking related to substance use behaviors and relapse.

CBT can be utilized at multiple levels (individual, couple, family or group) and in a variety of settings (inpatient, residential and outpatient levels of care).

Cognitive behavioral therapies for substance use include a range of interventions include

i. Contingency management
ii. Social/Coping skills training,
iii. Behavioral self-control training and
iv. Relapse prevention strategies.

i. Contingency Management

Contingency management (CM) is a behavioral shaping approach that provides tangible reinforcement (reward) for behaviors that reduce or illuminate substance use behaviors and prevent (maintaining abstinence or attending treatment activities . Research outcomes confirmed the effectiveness of (CM) strategies [4, 5].

Voucher-Based Reinforcement (VBR) and Prize Incentive Contingency management provide material reinforcement for drug-free urine test. The value of the voucher increases with consecutive negative drug screens [6].

ii. Social/Coping Skills Training

A primary goal of coping skills training is to help the individual develop and employ coping skills that effectively deal with the demands of high-risk situations without having to resort to substances as an alternative response [7].

A number of published treatment manuals are available to guide skills training with substance users. These manuals provide a session-by-session overview of the intervention. The skills to be taught are either specific to substance use (*e.g.*, coping with craving, refusing an offer of alcohol or drugs) or apply to more general interpersonal and emotional areas (*e.g.*, communication skills, coping with anger or depression). The functional analysis is of importance in determining the coping skills that should be addressed in this phase of treatment.

iii. Behavioral Self-Control Training

Behavioral Self-Control Training (BSCT) goal is harm reduction through decreased use. This approached can be self-directed or with the assistance of a therapist. Modern technology like computer software and applications can be of value [8, 9].

The technique is based on the following sequential steps:

1. Goal setting: Determine a maximum number of drinks per day.
2. Self-monitoring: Monitoring of the pattern of use (*e.g.*, how much, when,

where, with whom, feelings).

3. Rate control: reduce the amount consumed per target goal.
4. Drink refusal: develop assertiveness skills to refuse offered substances.
5. Rewarding goal attainment: develop reinforcement schedule when target goals are realized.
6. Functional analysis of drinking situations: functional analysis is an important tool that allows a map of emotional, social and environmental variables that promote use/none use of the substance.
7. Develop alternative coping skills other than use.
8. Relapse prevention training: see below.

iv. Relapse Prevention

Substance use disorders are chronic relapsing conditions, and relapses are common occurrences through the course of the illness. Relapse prevention goal is to build strategies to prevent relapses and reduce their impact and duration [10, 11].

Relapse prevention strategies include various components

1. **Develop a specific practical emergency plan in case of relapse:** Identify a list of accessible persons invested in the client's sobriety, best method to contact them in case help . Engage friends or family members in developing the emergency plan as their feedback about warning signs can be valuable.
2. **Develop coping strategies to deal with high risk situations:** see above, the techniques may include gradual exposure therapy to triggers of use.
3. **Healthy life balance:** achieving a better equilibrium, through pleasant activities and healthy life style has a value in reducing the impact of the stressors, Ineffective coping strategies and unbalanced life style gradually push the individuals closer to relapse.
4. **Cognitive Restructuring:** Negative cognitive schemas represent an organized pattern (think of an operating system software) of thoughts that organizes categories of information (experiences, memories, bodily sensations, emotions, cognitions, Behaviors) and the relationships among them, . Schemas are stable and generalized patterns, and once activated intense emotions are felt. As Clients experience relapse, schemas of hopelessness, helplessness and loss of

control are usually activated, generating a belief that relapse is internal (caused by one's defects) stable and generalized. In cognitive structuring the therapist helps the patient in shedding the light on these negative schemas and in identifying more rational attributions and relations (relapse is induced by a trigger (External) and the patient had insufficient training or practice on coping skills), (unstable and modifiable variable), Schemas related to positive expectations of drug use may also be restructured with the same principal.

Community Reinforcement Approach

The goal of this intervention is to increase the likelihood of continued abstinence from alcohol or drugs by structuring the patient's environment through a weakening of the influence of the reinforcement received by substance abuse and its related activities.

Reinforcement derived from healthier activities, like vocational, family, social, and recreational activities that are incompatible with substance abuse are strengthened. There is significant research proving the efficacy and effectiveness of this method.

Community reinforcement approach is based on providing positive reinforcement in sobriety rather than punishment in continued abuse. This modality has different components that are flexible which can be tailored to the needs of the individual.

Vocational counseling and job clubs, social and recreational counseling, marital counseling, and communication skills training are provided to enhance the quality of life and personal relationships [12, 13].

(AA), and several others. They are all patterned after the AA principles and involve acceptance, surrender to a higher power, and self-governance.

Motivational Interviewing

Several meta-analyses of motivational interview have shown strong evidence of efficacy in reducing substance use rates with durable effects lasing for several years in some individuals [14]. Motivational interviewing and motivation enhancement strategies are described in Chapter Six.

Solution-Focused Therapy

The solution-focused therapist believes that helping clients with substance use disorders through addressing any significant life problem can help them reduce their substance use. It is important to help the client find solutions to their problems while reinforcing the client's success in solving those problems. This procedure helps the client to recognize his/her own ability to solve problems. One technique of solution-focused therapy is to emphasize the exceptions to the client's problems. For example, the therapist directs the client's attention to periods of being substance-free. To identify these periods, the therapist listens to the client's responses and asks the client to elaborate on those periods with the purpose to help the client realize that he/she can maintain sobriety and has, in fact, done so in the past, and in many cases this period may have lasted months or years [15 - 17].

American Society of Addiction Medicine (ASAM) Placement Criteria

The American Society of Addiction Medicine created a model for substance use disorder evaluation with the goal of determining the required level of care (ASAM Placement Criteria -ASAM PPC-2R) [18].

The Model is Based on Assessing 6 Dimensions

i. Acute Intoxication and/or Withdrawal Potential

Assessing the needs of acutely intoxicated patients, planning for subsequent detoxification and withdrawal management.

ii. Biomedical Conditions and Complications

Evaluating the current medical problems and providing necessary care either within the current level of care or arranging and coordinating care with other health care providers.

iii. Emotional, Behavioral or Cognitive Conditions and Complications

Evaluating mental health issues and treating the condition within the provided level of care or coordinating and arranging for care with other health providers.

iv. Readiness to Change

Assessing patients motivation to treatment, and provide motivational enhancement strategies to advance towards treatment goals.

v. Relapse, Continued Use or Continued Problem Potential

Substance use disorders are chronic relapsing conditions that require active long term engagement, a continuum of interventions corresponding to the patients' stage of use, including Motivational enhancement, Harm reduction, Education and relapse prevention.

vi. Recovery Environment

Evaluate social circumstances that may affect treatment and influence sobriety or relapse as housing, social and family support, financial difficulties, occupational, educational, legal, access to transportation, social and childcare services.

Treatment Interventions are Organized in Gradually Increasing Intensity and Frequency Levels of Care

i. Early Intervention

Evaluation and education for individuals at risk of developing substance use disorders Ex:- (Hazardous use of alcohol)

ii. Outpatient Services

Level one includes outpatient care needs that are less than 9 hours of service/week for adults and less than 6 hours/week (adolescents).

iii. Intensive Outpatient: Includes the Following Subcategories

iii.i. Intensive Outpatient

Outpatient care that include or exceed 9 or more hours of service/week for (adults) and 6 or more hours/week (adolescents).

iii.ii. Partial Hospitalization

20 or more hours but less than 24 hours of service/week.

iv. Clinically-Managed Low-Intensity Residential

iv.i. Clinically-Managed Low-Intensity Residential

24 hour structure with trained personnel; clinical services are provided 5 hours or more per week

iv.ii. Clinically-Managed Medium-Intensity Residential

24 hour care with trained counselors

iv.iii. Clinically-Managed High-Intensity Residential

24 hour care with trained counselors to stabilize multidimensional imminent danger and prepare for outpatient treatment. Able to tolerate and use full active milieu or therapeutic community

iv.iv. Medically-Monitored Intensive Inpatient

24 hour nursing care with physician availability to address medical, psychiatric and withdrawal care needs

v. Medically-Managed Intensive Inpatient

24 hour nursing care and daily physician care for severe, unstable problems in Dimensions 1, 2 or 3. Counseling available to engage patient in treatment.

SUMMARY

Non-pharmacological evidenced-based behavioral interventions for substance use disorders are effective and are comparable to interventions for other psychiatric disorders [19].

COGNITIVE-BEHAVIORAL THERAPY AND OTHER PSYCHOSOCIAL INTERVENTIONS-PATIENT EDUCATION SHEET

What are the Behavioral Interventions for Substance Use Disorder?

Amongst others these include cognitive-behavioral therapy to help modify your thinking about reward driven repeated use of drugs or alcohol with talk therapy and/or reward-based treatment. In addition, time-tested 12-step Alcohol Anonymous (AA) based self-help groups are very valuable.

How Do these Work?

These help you by enhancing your ability to monitor external and internal cues and triggers and to use learned coping strategies and self-efficaciousness to deal with these and to prevent relapse.

How Effective are these?

Research shows that their efficacy is comparable to medications.

Who can Provide these Therapies?

Discuss this with your physician who may recommend a trained therapist in your community. Individuals in the 12-step fellowship may also make a recommendation.

Where can I Get More Information?

This can be obtained from following web site:

www.drugabuse.gov; www.niaaa.nih.gov

CONFLICT OF INTEREST

The authors confirm that they have no conflict of interest to declare for this publication.

ACKNOWLEDGEMENTS

Thanks to Sarit Hovav MD, for her review and constructive input to improve the quality of this manuscript.

REFERENCES

[1] Wilson B. Alcoholics Anonymous. Alcoholics Anonymous 1957.

[2] Ferri M, Amato L, Davoli M. Alcoholics Anonymous and other 12-step programmes for alcohol dependence. Cochrane Database Syst Rev 2006; 3(3): CD005032.
[PMID: 16856072]

[3] American Psychiatric Association. Position Statement on Substance Use Disorders 2012.

[4] Prendergast M, Podus D, Finney J, Greenwell L, Roll J. Contingency management for treatment of substance use disorders: a meta-analysis. Addiction 2006; 101(11): 1546-60.
[http://dx.doi.org/10.1111/j.1360-0443.2006.01581.x] [PMID: 17034434]

[5] Budney AJ, Moore BA, Rocha HL, Higgins ST. Clinical trial of abstinence-based vouchers and cognitive-behavioral therapy for cannabis dependence. J Consult Clin Psychol 2006; 74(2): 307-16.
[http://dx.doi.org/10.1037/0022-006X.74.2.307] [PMID: 16649875]

[6] Petry NM, Peirce JM, Stitzer ML, *et al.* Effect of prize-based incentives on outcomes in stimulant abusers in outpatient psychosocial treatment programs: a national drug abuse treatment clinical trials network study. Arch Gen Psychiatry 2005; 62(10): 1148-56.
[http://dx.doi.org/10.1001/archpsyc.62.10.1148] [PMID: 16203960]

[7] Kahan M, Wilson L, Becker L. Effectiveness of physician-based interventions with problem drinkers: a review. CMAJ 1995; 152(6): 851-9.
[PMID: 7697578]

[8] Hester RK, Delaney HD. Behavioral Self-Control Program for Windows: results of a controlled clinical trial. J Consult Clin Psychol 1997; 65(4): 686-93.
[http://dx.doi.org/10.1037/0022-006X.65.4.686] [PMID: 9256570]

[9] Miller WR, Muñoz RF. Controlling your drinking: tools to make moderation work for you. Guilford Press 2013.

[10] Annis HM, Davis CS. Relapse prevention training: A cognitive-behavioral approach based on self-efficacy theory. J Chem Depend Treat 1988; 2(2): 81-103.

[11] Bowen S, Chawla N, Marlatt GA. Mindfullness-based relapse prevention for treatment of substance use disorders: a clinician's guide. New York: Guilford Press 2010.

[12] Higgins ST. The influence of alternative reinforcers on cocaine use and abuse: a brief review. Pharmacol Biochem Behav 1997; 57(3): 419-27.
[http://dx.doi.org/10.1016/S0091-3057(96)00446-7] [PMID: 9218266]

[13] Miller WR, Meyers RJ, Hiller-Sturmhöfel S. The community-reinforcement approach. Alcohol Res Health 1999; 23(2): 116-21.
[PMID: 10890805]

[14] Hettema J, Steele J, Miller WR. Motivational interviewing. Annu Rev Clin Psychol 2005; 1: 91-111.
[http://dx.doi.org/10.1146/annurev.clinpsy.1.102803.143833] [PMID: 17716083]

[15] Monti PM, Rohsenow DJ, Swift RM, *et al.* Naltrexone and cue exposure with coping and communication skills training for alcoholics: treatment process and 1-year outcomes. Alcohol Clin Exp Res 2001; 25(11): 1634-47.
[http://dx.doi.org/10.1111/j.1530-0277.2001.tb02170.x] [PMID: 11707638]

[16] Donovan DM, Wells EA. 'Tweaking 12-Step': the potential role of 12-Step self-help group involvement in methamphetamine recovery. Addiction 2007; 102(s1) (Suppl. 1): 121-9.
[http://dx.doi.org/10.1111/j.1360-0443.2007.01773.x] [PMID: 17493061]

[17] Irvin JE, Bowers CA, Dunn ME, Wang MC. Efficacy of relapse prevention: a meta-analytic review. J Consult Clin Psychol 1999; 67(4): 563-70.
[http://dx.doi.org/10.1037/0022-006X.67.4.563] [PMID: 10450627]

[18] Mee-Lee D, Shulman GD. "The ASAM Placement Criteria and Matching Patients to Treatment". Chapter 27 in Section 4. Overview of Addiction Treatment. In: Eds:Ries RK, Miller S, Fiellin DA, Saitz R, Eds. Principles of Addiction Medicine. Fourth Edition. Philadelphia PA: Lippincott Williams & Wilkins 2009; pp. 387-99.

[19] Dutra L, Stathopoulou G, Basden SL, Leyro TM, Powers MB, Otto MW. A meta-analytic review of psychosocial interventions for substance use disorders. Am J Psychiatry 2008; 165(2): 179-87.
[http://dx.doi.org/10.1176/appi.ajp.2007.06111851] [PMID: 18198270]

SUBJECT INDEX

A

B

C

D

E

F

K

L

M

P

Q

R

S

T

U

V

W

www.ingramcontent.com/pod-product-compliance
Lightning Source LLC
LaVergne TN
LVHW070935210926
848482LV00003B/241